# HEALTH PERSONNEL

## Meeting the Explosive Demand for Medical Care

by Harold M. Goldstein
Morris A. Horowitz
with the assistance of
Kathleen A. Calore

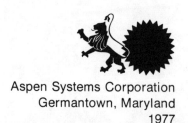

Aspen Systems Corporation
Germantown, Maryland
1977

Library of Congress Catalog Card Number: 76-55042
ISBN: 0-912862-36-X

*Printed in the United States of America.*

3  4  5

Typesetting by Howard Kirshen Printing Corp., Boston, MA.

To

Michelle, Debora

Carol and Ruth

This study was funded by the Office of Research and Development Education and Training Administration, United States Department of Labor. This study does not necessarily represent the official opinion or policy of the Employment and Training Administration or Northeastern University. The authors are solely responsible for the contents of the study.

# Contents

# Tables

# Acknowledgments

This study began in March 1974 and ran concurrently with several ongoing projects at the Center for Medical Manpower Studies of the Economics Department at Northeastern University. The basic concept of this project developed from a challenge by Dr. Howard Rosen, Director, Office of Research and Development, Employment and Training Administration, U.S. Department of Labor, to document whether the well-publicized decrease in hospital occupancy rates in 1974 would have any short- and long-range impacts on the quantity and variety of health manpower employed by health providers. We accepted the challenge, and the project was funded by that office.

We are indebted to a large number of people who gave freely of their time and ideas. To Dr. Rosen we owe our greatest thanks for his ideas, encouragement, and support. We owe a special thanks to Mr. William Throckmorton, Project Monitor, and to others of the Office of Research and Development who were extremely helpful in designing the research plan and in conducting the work.

We wish to thank a large number of persons who assisted the Center in gathering local, state, and national data. They include: John Brewer, Massachusetts Department of Public Health; John R. Dinkelspiel, Chairman, Task Force on Allied Health Manpower, Massachusetts Office of Manpower Affairs; Edward R.

Donovan, Director of Massachusetts Rate Setting Commission, Bureau of Hospitals; Paul Von Ebers, Project Director, Division of Survey Research, American Hospital Association, E. Martin Egelston, Director, Bureau of Research Services, American Hospital Association; Louis Freedman, Acting Director, Office of Health Planning and Statistics, Massachusetts Department of Public Health; David Gagnon, Associate Director of Planning, Massachusetts Office of Comprehensive Health Planning, Executive Office of Human Services; Ernest Henderson, Chairman, Research and Development Committee, Massachusetts Federation of Nursing Homes, Henderson Houses of America; Ralph C. Kuhli, Director, Department of Allied Medical Professions and Services, American Medical Association; John J. Lennon, Director, Bureau of Nursing Homes, Rest Homes and Convalescent Homes, Massachusetts Rate Setting Commission; Philip McCarthy, Research Associate, Department of Allied Medical Professions and Services, American Medical Association; Richard Olsen, Director of Education, Massachusetts General Hospital; E. Elizabeth Swenson, Allied Health Task Force, Office of Manpower Affairs; Harold Wallach, Social Research Consultant.

In addition we are indebted to many people who were directly involved in gathering statistical information for this study from their own institutions. They include Jocelyn Allen, Administrator, Faulkner Hospital; Robert Bass, Personnel Director, Veterans Administration Hospital, West Roxbury; Robert Bauer, Personnel Director, Massachusetts Rehabilitation Hospital; Regina Brooks, Administrator, New England Sinai Hospital; Melvin Cohen, M.D., Administrator, Glenside Hospital; Wallace Countze, Deputy Commissioner of Personnel, Boston City Hospital; Allen DesRosiers, Assistant Administrator, Sancta Maria Hospital; William Donovan, Administrator, Youville Hospital; Samuel B. Edelstein, Beth Israel Hospital; Stanley M. Fertel, Executive Director, Jewish Memorial Hospital; William W. Feuer, Associate Director, Peter Bent Brigham Hospital; D. Frances Frassa, Personnel Director, The Cambridge Hospital; Betsy Ray Fuller, Personnel Director, Boston Hospital for Women; Bruce Hadley, Personnel Director, Longwood Hospital;

Thomas J. Hogan, Personnel Officer, Veterans Administration Hospital, Jamaica Plain; Barbara Hooker, Personnel Director, Kennedy Memorial Hospital for Children; Lynn A. Houston, Manager of Employment Services, St. Elizabeth's Hospital; Fay Kaufman, Personnel Director, Mt. Auburn Hospital; Robert Lallesie, Personnel Director, Massachusetts Mental Health Center; M. Marinelli, Personnel Director, Harley Private Hospital; C.C. Marino, M.D., Medical Director, Kenmore Hospital; Rita S. McDonough, Director of Employee Relations and Administrative Services, Robert B. Brigham Hospital; Sally Mokrash, Personnel Director, Hahnemann Hospital; Michael Nelson, M.D., Superintendent, Boston State Hospital; Suzanne Persky, Senior Personnel Assistant, Massachusetts Eye and Ear Infirmary; Thomas Reichard, Personnel Director, St. Margaret's Hospital; Elizabeth Sheehy, Director of Nurses, Shriners Burns Institute; David Tedesco, Employment and Employee Benefits Administrator, Hebrew Rehabilitation Center for the Aged; Viola Thacker, Personnel Director, Lemuel Shattuck Hospital; Richard Thurm, M.D., Administrator, U.S. Public Health Service Hospital.

For information on ambulatory center and other health providers we are indebted to Chester A. Alper, M.D., Center for Blood Research; Stephen Baran, ABCD/Columbia Point Health Center; Robert Batal, East Boston Neighborhood Health Center; Mrs. Bender, Douglas A. Thom Clinic for Children; Mr. Black, South End Community Health Center; Ms. Beswick, University of Massachusetts, Columbia Point; Richard J. Cannon, Cambridge Center, Harvard Community Health Plan; Dwight Conrad, Neighborhood Family Care Center; Deborah Demy, Cambridge-Somerville Mental Health Center; Gloria Desrochers, Northeastern University; Ms. Donahue, Commercial Union Clinic; Dr. Duda, Cambridge Day Center; Mrs. Halley, Visiting Nurse Association of Cambridge; Ms. Herrick, Crittenton-Hastings House Clinic; Mrs. Hollinger, Cambridge Guidance Center; Howard Hoople, Project Place Emergency Services; Penelope Hope, Visiting Nurse Association of Boston; Margaret Ives, Harvard Community Health Plan; Donald Johnson,

Dimock Community Health Center; Elizabeth LaCamera, East Boston-Winthrop Clinic; Mr. Landry, Family Service Association of Greater Boston; Janis MacMillan, South End Health Unit; William Manzakas, Martha Eliot Health Center; Mr. Moore, Whittier Street Health Center; Charles F. Mullen, O.D., Massachusetts College of Optometry; Ms. O'Donnell, Overholt Thoracic Clinic; Barbara Nas, South Boston Court Clinic; William Quinn, Tufts University School of Dental Medicine; Gener Thompson, Department of Community Medicine, The Cambridge Hospital; Howard Veit, Mission Hill-Parker Hill Clinic; James L. Wells, Roxbury Court Clinic; and Mrs. Williams, Forsyth Dental Infirmary for Children.

A special thanks to all those who conducted the on-site visits and interviews to collect data—Patricia McCarville, John N. Burns, Farhoud Kafi-Tehrani, and Robert Vinson. We also wish to acknowledge the assistance of those who verified and coded this data—Christine Cormier, Michael Shelby, and Kerry Bogle.

The preparation and typing of the numerous preparatory tables and of the final manuscript of this report were done by Sylvia Goldberg, Rosalie Hausserman, Alec Cheloff, Patricia McCarville, and Bonnie Campbell. The manuscript was edited by Diane Ullius Jarrett and Pauline Simons. Lila and Debora Goldstein assisted in the proofreading and indexing process. Their assistance in these chores is hereby acknowledged.

The views and judgments of this study are ours alone and do not represent those of our consultants or their institutions, the health providers included in this study, or the Employment and Training Administration. All who assisted in this project undoubtedly contributed in giving this study whatever success it has. We alone bear the responsibility for the complete study, including the conclusions and recommendations as well as the errors of omission and commission.

# HEALTH
# PERSONNEL

# 1

## Introduction

It has generally been assumed, wisely or not, that the health care industry has the unlimited capacity to expand and absorb large numbers of health care personnel. This assumption has led to substantial increases in training programs for various allied health occupations and to a rapidly growing supply of persons who consider themselves affiliated with the health care industry.

This notion of growth has been based largely on the fact that over the past decade there has been a significant increase in the number of new hospitals, adding substantial numbers of beds and highly sophisticated specialty facilities, such as cobalt therapy and intensive and cardiac care units. These developments were fueled by the monies provided by the federal government, specifically under the Hill-Burton Act, Medicare, and Medicaid.

In this report we will assess the concept of growth of the health industry. The previous expansion of facilities gives little assurance that growth will continue or that utilization of existing facilities is at levels that can be considered economical.

The following questions are addressed in this report:

1. Is there an excess bed capacity in hospitals now? What is the trend?

2. If the occupancy rate is declining, is there a real need to expand the supply of various categories of health care manpower?

3. If part of the decline in the hospital occupancy rate is due to a shift from inpatient to outpatient care, what is the impact on employment in various health care occupations and in the industry as a whole?

4. To what extent has the introduction of new types of providers of health care services—such as extended care facilities, neighborhood health centers, and health maintenance organizations—changed the demand, structure, and utilization of health care personnel?

5. What are the major employment trends in the categories of health personnel employed by traditional health care providers (hospitals) and by new types of providers?

Before discussing health manpower, it is important to describe the scene in which these workers function. First we will present a brief review of health trends and of major health indicators. We will then describe the health occupations and the problems of utilization.

## Health Trends

From 1900 to 1950 modern medicine in the United States had an enormous positive impact on the effects of disease through improvements that alleviated suffering, eradicated many severe illnesses, prevented crippling, and postponed untimely death. These changes have been closely associated with higher standards of living, better housing, and improved educational opportunities. Such drugs as penicillin provide immediate cures for such diseases as lobar pneumonia, which decades ago claimed one-quarter of its victims.

The most valid indices of health status are life expectancy and infant mortality. Life expectancy is a theoretical annual estimate of the average life expectancy of a newborn; it reflects the probabilities of illness during one's lifetime. The infant mortality rate is the number of infants who die in the first year of life out of every 1,000 live births. Infant mortality is a prime indicator of the effectiveness of the health care system, since the availability of proper care has an almost immediate impact on the survival rate of infants through proper prenatal and obstetrical care, as do better nutrition and increased supervision during the first year of life.

As a result of advances during the first half of the twentieth century, there was a decrease in infant mortality and a general increase in life expectancy. However, despite the enormous expansion of medical facilities, expenditures on medical research, and increases in health manpower in the subsequent twenty-five years, there has been a steady leveling off in health progress. Dr. David Rutstein of the Harvard Medical School described this enormous expansion of medical research, facilities, and manpower together with our lagging national health picture as the paradox of modern medicine in the United States.[1]

Between 1965 and 1972 expenditures on health care in the United States skyrocketed from $39.0 billion to $89.5 billion, representing an increase from 5.9 percent to 7.7 percent of the gross national product (GNP). Per capita expenditures on health care amounted to $422, up $43 (11.4 percent). In 1972 third-party payers met 90 percent of the hospital bill, 58 percent of physicians' bills, 13 percent of the bill for dental care and drugs, and 60 percent of the total spent for other services. Nevertheless there was an 8.5 percent increase in direct per capita payments over the 1971 figure.[2]

Despite these increases in expenditures and costs, the United States has failed to improve the health status of its population substantially over the past decade. The major health indices have shown very little improvement in recent years.

Although major health problems still vary from one country to another, the general health status has improved in most European nations over the past twenty years. Comparisons of some of the more industrial nations of Europe with the United States demonstrate that most of them have made significant progress in improving the quality of care while the United States has not made much headway. In the European nations there has been a continuous decline in infant mortality rates and a lengthening of average life expectancy at birth. The distribution of population by age has shifted so that those over 60 years of age account for more than 15 percent and, in some cases, 20 percent of the population.[3]

However, the most outstanding improvement in health status has been in the younger age groups. The median infant mortality rate in European nations decreased from 30 to about 20 per 1,000 live births between 1962 and 1972.[4] In great measure these decreases are due directly to the significant rise in the number and utilization of allied health personnel.

In the first half of this century the United States made consistent progress in lengthening the life expectancy of its citizens. In 1920 the expectation of life at birth for the total population was 54.1 years; by 1960 the figure had increased to 69.7 years.[5] However, this trend has slowed to a near standstill. The figure for 1972 indicates an expectation of life of only 71.2 years, an increase of a mere 2.1 percent over the 1960 figure.[6]

Only two of the ten countries listed in table 32 (Ch. 6) have infant mortality rates higher than that of the United States. The United States also maintained the highest inpatient admission rate (1,611 per 10,000 population) of the ten countries. The average length of hospital stay for the United States was the lowest of the reporting countries; at the same time this country had the highest population per bed (130) and the lowest overall occupancy rate (78 percent).

## Major Health Indicators

Numerous health indicators exist, but it is generally accepted that there are five major indicators.

### The Growth of Health Expenditures

Health care expenditures grew from 4.6 percent of the GNP in 1940 to 5.3 percent of the GNP in 1960.[7] By 1970 they were $69.2 billion, or 7.1 percent of the GNP, and in 1975 the estimated figure rose to $115 billion, or about 8 percent of the GNP.[8] Projections for 1980 indicate health care expenditures could rise to 10 percent of the GNP.[9]

## Death Rates and Infant Mortality Rates

According to the United Nations *Statistical Yearbook, 1974*, of the seventy countries listing crude death rates in 1968, forty-four had lower death rates and ten had lower infant mortality rates than the United States. In 1972 the U.S. nonwhite death rates for both the general population and infants were nearly twice those of the white race.

## Hospital Facilities and Health Personnel

Between 1963 and 1973 the number of hospital beds in the United States failed to keep pace with the increase in population. The population per hospital bed increased from 110.7 in 1963 to 136.1 in 1973..In fact, of 206 countries listing hospital beds per capita in the United Nations *Statistical Yearbook, 1974*, 44 had more beds per capita than the United States.

In 1960 the estimated number of persons employed in various occupations in the health field represented 3.7 percent of the urban labor force; by 1970 the percentage had increased to 4.7 percent. The federal health manpower training budget increased by 54 percent from 1969 to 1974 ($717 to $1,101 million in constant dollars);[10] health professional employment increased 47 percent while the share of minority employment more than doubled. The numbers of active health professionals per 100,000 population have increased steadily during the 1950-74 period.[11]

## Geographic Distribution of Facilities and Manpower

In 1972 the average number of beds per 1,000 population in the United States was 7.4; the rate ranged from 5.3 beds in New Hampshire to 19.6 beds in the District of Columbia. In 1972 the United States averaged 160 active physicians per 100,000 population, but the figures ranged from 92 in Mississippi to 242 in New York State. The national average of registered nurses per 100,000 population was 382, ranging from 227 in Mississippi to 581 in Connecticut. The geographic distribution of health manpower continues to be uneven; the East-South Central states have only about half as many physicians, dentists, and nurses relative to the population as the Middle Atlantic or the New England states.[12] This maldistribution will not be easily reversed, because higher income states will continue to attract health workers in large numbers.

## The Ability to Pay the Cost of Medical Care

Preliminary figures for 1974 show that the average per capita income in the United States was $5,434, ranging from $3,764 in Mississippi to $7,023 in Alaska. However, even the per capita income in Mississippi was surpassed by only eight out of eighty-five countries listing per capita income in the United Nations *Statistical Yearbook, 1974.*[13]

Within the past six years (1969 through 1974) there has been a rapid expansion in the nation's expenditures for health and related activities. The growth of federal health expenditures has kept pace with the growth of total health spending, the former accounting for approximately twenty-six cents of the national health dollar over the period. Federal health expenditures have increased more rapidly than the federal budget as a whole and now account for 12 percent of the budget, compared with only 9 percent in 1969.[14]

The last decade has been a period of increased federal financial commitment in the health sector. The nature of federal involvement in the health care system has changed considerably, however; the most significant area of growth was in the legislation providing funds for two health care programs. The Medicare program—introduced in 1967 for the elderly—and, later, the Medicaid system for those in financial need accounted for 56 percent of the federal health financial commitment in 1974. The total federal expenditure increased from $4.6 billion in 1967 to $18.0 billion in 1974 (in current dollars).[15]

Over the past decade Americans have increasingly taken advantage of private health insurance plans covering in-hospital and surgical expenditures. By 1970 approximately 80 percent of all Americans were covered by private and public insurance plans; two decades earlier the figure had been less than half the population. The enactment of the Medicare program covered 21 million Americans with public insurance. The addition of Medicaid further underwrote the cost of medical care for the indigent. Despite this substantial progress in health insurance coverage, it is estimated that 20 to 40 million people in the United States are without any health insurance coverage whatsoever.[16]

## Terminology

In order to understand all the ramifications of this study, it is important to define some of the key terms used. What is meant by health personnel? What is meant by a shortage or surplus within a single occupation? Who are the professionals in the industry?

As in many industries of our market economy, the personnel in the health care industry ranges from the unskilled to the professional. However, there is no general agreement in the health industry as to who are the professionals and who come under other broad classifications. Fifty years ago it seemed clear that physicians (and probably dentists and pharmacists) were the only professionals of the industry. As a result of growth and changes in the last thirty years, there is considerable uncertainty as to which occupations are to be considered professional and what distinctions, if any, should be made among the numerous classifications that are not considered professional.

To some the term *professional* is restricted to the physician alone, since it is the only occupation in the industry that requires a bachelor's degree plus medical school training. This nicely fits the dictionary definition of the learned professions of theology, law, and medicine. However, in order to classify the numerous other occupations in the industry, such terms as *paraprofessional, subprofessional, semiprofessional, paramedical,* and *auxiliary* have

been developed. But these terms have no consistent pattern of
usage. Because of conflicting applications these terms have caused
confusion and occasional bitterness among various groups in the
industry. By some definitions the term *paraprofessional* (or paramedical) includes registered nurses, sanitary engineers, radiologic
technologists and technicians, and even veterinarians and dentists. The terms *auxiliary* and *ancillary* have been used by some to
describe a broad category of workers who are considered to be dis-
tinctly subordinate to the professional and paramedical categories. The term *subprofessional* has caused most problems,
because of the connotation of the word. It tends to diminish the
status of the groups it encompasses, and it could inhibit the development of a sense of responsibility in the employees of occupations so classified.

Many health occupational groups have organized themselves
into unions and professional associations, and they consider
themselves to be professional, although they could hardly meet
the time-honored definition of "theology, law, and medicine."
Certainly many so-called professional groups in the United States
function as highly structured organizations that have key interests in certification and accreditation requirements, although
some groups would not meet any rigid criterion of graduate education, undergraduate education or, in some instances, even a
high school diploma.

By sheer numbers the registered nurse (RN) now plays an important role among health providers, but there is no unanimity on
whether the nurse is a professional. In some instances the RN
might have a master's degree, in a larger number of cases, a bachelor of science degree. Typically, however, the nurse is a graduate
of a three-year program, and graduates of two-year programs are
still quite common. Is the principal criterion for classification a
license or certification that specifies a minimum level of education? Or are the duties and functions performed the key to the classification? Again, there is no agreed-upon answer. However, at
this point, it should be noted that there is tremendous overlap in
the performance of medical functions among all levels of health
personnel, from the physician through the registered nurse to the

entry-level health employee, and nearly all may consider themselves professional.

An example of the problem is the electrocardiographic (EKG) or electroencephalographic (EEG) technician, who performs a full range of medical functions. In numerous instances a person in this classification may have a secondary school education (in some cases, even less) but may have been trained on the job in the hospital by a cardiologist. After some years of experience in such a position, the average EKG or EEG technician is likely to consider him/herself a professional. By what standards does one classify these positions as subprofessional or paraprofessional?

During and immediately after World War II it was common to classify most health care occupations, save the physician, as paramedical personnel. This term included all health care occupations from the registered nurse to the entry-level medical or surgical nursing aides. During the late 1960s the term *paramedical personnel* fell into disrepute, principally because many in the occupations felt the term debased their "professional" image and prestige. The word *paramedical* was replaced by the phrase *allied health*. The striving for status and recognition by various occupation groups soon brought about the rejection of *allied*; there was a desire to be independent and not attached to any specific subgroup or occupation. By 1975 there seemed to be a strong move to adopt the term *health personnel* to cover all occupations related to health, including the physician.

In view of these changes this report will use the terms *allied health* or *health personnel* or occupation, with no intention of slighting or disparaging any occupation or group. Our interest is to include all those persons in the industry who relate directly to the patient—"laying hands on." The terms used are intended to cover the whole range of health workers, from physicians and physician extenders (such as pediatric nurse practitioners and graduate registered nurses with four or five years of formal schooling after secondary school) to the entry-level nurse's aide or assistant (NA) and the laboratory assistant who may have less than a high school education plus on-the-job training, in-service education, or both. The physician is included, not because this profession is our prime focus but because of the key relationships between it and many of the other classifications in the industry.

As late as 1910 there were essentially only three members of the health care team—physician, nurse, and aide. By 1974 the figure rose to well over 450 individual health care occupations.[17] The most current estimate puts the figure at 600,[18] but this total undoubtedly includes some health occupations that are listed more than once under different job titles. Nonetheless, it is impossible to classify the range of titles accurately into professional and entry-level positions.

In the same fashion, there is no agreement as to which classifications may be considered ports of entry for the unskilled and untrained. In some hospitals and in some geographic areas, certain occupations are considered entry-level; with experience and training on the job, the employees are moved up an occupational ladder. There is no uniform industry pattern of hiring-in occupations or of moving up a ladder. The occupation of surgical technician may be cited as an example. In most instances the surgical technician was first employed by the health provider in an entry-level occupation, such as nurse's aide. She or he could have functioned as a nurse's aide for several months or a year before being assigned to the surgery department. It is not unusual for individuals in entry-level jobs to be exposed to on-the-job training or inservice education programs in the department of surgery, where the training is provided by staff surgeons. At some point in the training the person may be classified as a surgical technician. This situation is typical in the United States Navy, where after two or three years of on-the-job training an entry-level aide finds himself as a functioning member of a surgical team. There is no uniform pattern in the industry of hiring in, of training, or of promotion.

## General Characteristics of Health Workers

When discussing the possibility of a shortage of health manpower, do we assume that there are numerous local labor markets and that the employees do not migrate readily from one market to another? Or is there a single national labor market, and are health manpower personnel very mobile on a national scale? Is a surplus of RNs or NAs measured solely in terms of unemployed persons with specific qualifications? What are the implications if RNs or NAs are able to perform the functions of LPNs, who are in short supply?

The problems of defining "shortage" become apparent in the discussion of three hospitals that have cooperated in the research efforts of the Center for Medical Manpower Studies. All are short-term, general hospitals of comparable size, but each is situated in a different geographical area and therefore faces different labor market conditions. One hospital is in rural Maine, another is in Boston, and the other is in New York City. The rural facility has little difficulty in staffing at all levels of skill because the hospital is the largest single employer in the area. Wage rates at all levels are approximately 25 percent lower than in Boston hospitals and 50 percent lower than in the hospitals of New York. The turnover rate at semiprofessional and professional levels in the Boston and New York hospitals was well above the rates at the rural hospital. The current period of high unemployment has dampened the 100 to 150 percent turnover rates for entry-level personnel in the Boston and New York hospitals, but their rates are still high relative to those in the rural Maine hospital.

In 1967 a detailed study of health personnel in the greater Boston area by Professor Dean S. Ammer reached the following conclusions:[19]

1. Demand for allied health skills will outstrip the supply in the foreseeable future.

2. Institutions deal with shortages by relying on part-time or less skilled help and by providing inferior services.

3. Shortages are not uniformly distributed.

4. Wider pay differentials should be encouraged.

5. Status-hungry allied health organizations indirectly contribute to the shortages.

6. Allied health middle management is poorly trained in techniques of administration.

Dr. Eli Ginzberg of Columbia University made some pointed comments about the health manpower situation. He noted that in virtually all fields dependent on trained manpower there are complaints of shortages but that all will fail to meet their needs if they insist on perpetuating their old cumbersome patterns of staffing. Every field, including health care, finds the shifting of goals and redirection of resources difficult because of inflexibility, conservative attitudes, and weak leadership. He goes on to note that in a dynamic society time produces changes, and that the institutions brought into being at an earlier period to cope with particular problems have in fact been eroded by alterations in the environment and in the priority needs of the population. To cope with these problems, Ginzberg suggests such adjustments as eliminating or merging some tasks, reassigning tasks to personnel with less formal training and skills, substituting money for manpower in the performance of some functions, and transferring functions from the provider to the consumer of the service.[20]

In April 1973 the Committee for Economic Development published a report entitled *Building a National Health Care System,* which states:

Poor distribution, together with inadequate utilization, training, and organization, have aggravated the shortages of manpower in some areas while causing surpluses in others. Beyond some crude and increasingly doubtful ratios of professions to population, it is not even known how many people are now needed let alone how many would be needed under a better-organized system.[21]

If the market for health manpower operated efficiently without artificial barriers, supply and demand would ultimately correct shortages. Institutions would act to retain or attract employees, restructure hiring standards and pay scales, institute training programs, and explore new sources of recruitment. However, in the real world this has not happened. Hospitals have not moved adequately to correct high turnover rates, job dissatisfaction, relatively low wage levels, and limited upward mobility.

The actions of employers have been matched by the attitudes of some groups of health workers. As health workers become more specialized, they tend to seek a higher professional status and to mimic the exclusionary guild practices of the representative model—the physician.[22] As health occupations form their own interest groups, they further limit the mobility of workers without professional credentials.

The manpower shortages in the health care industry may be somewhat contrived by the institutions in the system, but it appears that shortages do exist and will continue through the 1970s. We note the following facts:

1. Wage rates for health personnel, though still below those of manufacturing employees, have increased over the last five years at a rate higher than the average for all workers.[23]

2. Even with the character of its services and the round-the-clock nature of the health industry, the attrition of the labor force appears abnormally high; for some occupations the training is barely keeping pace with the need for replacements.

3. The enormous growth of technical knowledge has fragmented the occupations of health workers. At the beginning of this century the physician, nurse, and aide were probably the only recognized categories of health workers. In 1974 no less than 425 specialty groups, other than physicians, were identified in the health care field. Advances in technology have expanded the labor-intensive nature of the health care industry. Thus, despite the fact that inpatient occupancy rates have remained relatively constant, the number of health workers employed by these same hospitals has been increasing substantially.

Excluding the physician, a substantial majority of the 4 million or more workers in the health labor force are employed in hospitals. A smaller number are employed by private practicing physicians, and a rather small minority are employed in nursing and rest homes and in private laboratories. It has been estimated that in 1973 over half of the health care employees were in low-income jobs paying about $4,000 a year, and that about 90 percent were women, 20 percent black.[24]

Although the wages of health care workers have shown rapid growth in the last decade, their earnings remain relatively low. Certainly one of the principal factors influencing the unstable work force, particularly in the lower level positions, is the disparity in wage scales.[25]

## The Problem of Excess Bed Capacity

In 1946 the Congress passed the Hill-Burton Act, which provided a program to deal with the shortage of hospitals that had developed during the Depression and World War II. Since then approximately $3.8 billion in Hill-Burton grants have been distributed to nearly 11,000 hospitals and other health facilities.

It was generally assumed that more hospital facilities would automatically result in better health care. The need for hospital beds was deemed especially acute in poor rural areas and in the South. However, new medical facilities have been financed and erected without any comprehensive regional or national plan. Physicians and boards of trustees of hospitals have decided that new facilities were desirable and then constructed these facilities, paying little attention to possible duplication or the real need for the facilities.

Following the example set by New York in 1965, twenty-three states have enacted laws requiring that hospitals obtain certificates of need before making any significant additions or erecting a new medical facility as an effort to remedy this situation. Certificates of need are usually granted by a state health officer with the concurrence of state and local planning agencies. Despite their apparent authority, certificate of need committees have not exercised their power strictly; as a result, more and more facilities continue to be expanded. Because boards of trustees frequently represent commercial interests (banks, insurance companies, and construction firms), there appears to be a vested interest in expanding medical facilities regardless of the needs of the community.

Physicians also may have a personal interest in expanding an existing facility or erecting a completely new hospital. As new equipment becomes available as a result of significant scientific and technological breakthroughs, hospitals build new facilities to accommodate it. Thus new medical facilities have sprung up in all parts of the nation, even in areas where the utilization rates were already at the breakeven point. It is generally accepted in the industry that an occupancy rate of 75 to 85 percent is necessary for a hospital to operate economically, yet a substantial number of hospitals are listed by the American Hospital Association as operating at a rate well below 80 percent.

For a number of years there has been growing concern about hospital underutilization and excess bed capacity. As a result the managers of Hill-Burton funds began stressing the modernization of outdated urban hospitals, rather than the construction of new facilities, and by 1971 only 4 percent of Hill-Burton funds were designated for new hospital construction. In addition, there has been increased recognition of the need for improved ambulatory services in hospitals.

If there is excess bed capacity in hospitals now, what is the trend, and what is the long-range projection? If the utilization rate is declining, is there a real need to expand the supply of health care manpower? And what will happen to the utilization of current health care personnel? If part of the decline in the hospital occupancy rate is due to a shift from inpatient to outpatient care, what is the impact on employment in different health occupations? To what extent has the introduction of new kinds of providers of health care services, such as extended care facilities, neighborhood health centers, and health maintenance organizations, changed the structure and utilization of health care personnel and perhaps even created a greater demand for certain occupations?

The expansion of technical knowledge in the medical field is an important factor in the demand for all health care manpower and new medical specialist occupations. Five decades ago the ratio of health employees to physician was approximately 4 to 1; at present the ratio is 12 to 1. Whatever the manpower results of excess bed capacity, they must be balanced against the changing relationship between physicians and other health workers.

In summary, the utilization of health personnel in the United States appears to have followed the following pattern:

1. Reports of manpower shortages in hospitals tend to reflect

an inflated number of budgeted positions, and not necessarily the need for qualified health workers. Indeed, even if skilled medical personnel had been available to fill vacancies, there is no guarantee that they would have been hired.

2. There has been a rather random, piecemeal effort to lower operating expenses by substituting lower level medical personnel, such as aides and technicians, for RNs, LPNs, and technologists.

3. Although the wages of health workers have increased substantially over the last decade, their earnings are still relatively low, despite widespread reports of manpower shortages.

4. The health industry over the last several decades has been characterized by factors that inhibit employment: high turnover rates, job dissatisfaction, and limited upward job mobility.

# 2

## Methodology

### Utilization of Health Manpower

The Center for Medical Manpower Studies (CMMS) at Northeastern University began the current research early in 1974 as an extension of its principal activities in the field of health manpower. The Center has been concerned with the problems of improving utilization of health workers, on the assumption that a shortage of such personnel (especially at the higher levels) existed.

The project was prompted by the question of whether there was any direct evidence of an expanding need for health personnel, in view of the decreasing occupancy rate in hospitals. Of course, the very concept of a shortage depended on the definition of the term. It is impossible to obtain a quick measure of shortage except by some proxy measure. The CMMS undertook to collect and analyze data on the employment of health workers in the Boston area during a five-year period in order to determine whether the decline in hospital utilization rates meant a real decline in the demand for health services and therefore a relative surplus rather than a shortage of health personnel.

Our original intent was to obtain health employment data for two years, 1967 and 1972, from the 250 principal employers of health personnel in Boston and Cambridge. Limiting the geographic scope to Boston and Cambridge seemed adequate in view of the high concentration of various types of health care facilities in these cities. The five-year span would provide an optimum period for studying any changes that might have occurred. It was determined by a brief pretest that data for before 1967 and after 1972 would be difficult to obtain.

Once work on this project began, it became apparent that there were no consistent and reliable sources of health manpower data on a local level or on state, regional, or national levels. Several other groups were concerned about this void and had begun to work to fill the gap. One such project was a study undertaken by a task force established by the Office of Manpower Affairs of the Commonwealth of Massachusetts (OMA). This project had developed a manpower questionnaire that was included in the *Annual (1973) Report* to the Massachusetts Department of Public Health (DPH), required of all nursing homes, rest homes, and ambulatory facilities. An arrangement was made between the DPH, the OMA, and the CMMS, whereby the CMMS would process and code the state's surveys in return for use of the information.

Since the OMA-DPH project had already distributed a questionnaire for the year 1973, the CMMS survey period was revised to cover the years 1968 through 1973. At the same time it was decided to include 1971 data, in order to pinpoint when various changes occurred.

Since the target of our research involved a wide variety of health facilities, including some private proprietary (for-profit) hospitals and nursing and rest homes, the preliminary steps were to secure information already collected before approaching facilities individually. At the outset of this project we anticipated that we would have the most difficulty in obtaining information from the proprietary nursing and rest homes.

The OMA-DPH survey of nursing and rest homes contained much of the needed 1973 employment data from 95 percent of these facilities throughout the state. The questionnaire had been distributed to these facilities as part of the required annual survey, which accounted for the extremely high response rate.

The OMA-DPH 1973 survey of ambulatory facilities was far less successful, but it did provide a starting point for our efforts in tracking down ambulatory centers. However, only half of all facilities responded; the poorest return was from those in the city of Boston. The CMMS staff contacted each facility in the Boston-Cambridge survey area, first by phone, then by mail (see Appendix A, Appendix B). Finally about seventy-five on-site visits were made to complete the survey. In general the ambulatory facilities were willing to cooperate, but the needed 1973 records often were not available, since many of the facilities were newly established.

In order to obtain data for 1968 and 1971 we contacted the Massachusetts Rate Setting Commission (RSC), a state agency that collects and audits the financial statements of hospitals and nursing and rest homes. The RSC-1 form, which all nursing and rest homes are required to complete annually, was invaluable in providing manpower data on the period studied. The dollar amount spent on salaries for the three major categories employed (RNs, LPNs, NAs) in these facilities is specified on this form. To make it possible to translate these figures into number of employees, the Rate Setting Commission provided an average hourly wage for these categories for 1968, 1971, and 1973. The dollar figures were converted into manhours, which were then translated into full-time equivalent (FTE) figures. The OMA-DPH survey data for 1973 corresponded closely to the FTEs calculated from the budget figures from the RSC-1 data.

The use of FTE figures was adopted in our methodology in order to adjust for the significant number of part-time workers in the health industry, particularly in nursing and rest homes. In our calculations each part-time worker was counted as one-half of a full-time worker. This estimate was confirmed by crosschecking the 1973 employment figures in 10 percent of the facilities in our survey against the staffing levels required by the state department of Public Health.

One of our concerns in this research has been the development of an ongoing system of data collection. Our involvement with the OMA-DPH 1973 survey provided us with examples of problems in survey design and thereby enriched our experience. We were also offered the opportunity to make suggestions for the 1975 OMA survey.

The data from hospitals within our survey area were the most difficult to collect. The hospital administrators and, in some cases, the personnel directors, were telephoned by the Center's director, who explained the project. We secured the promise of cooperation from all the hospitals in the Boston-Cambridge area, and every telephone call was followed up by a letter and a copy of our questionnaire.

Many facilities apparently fail to keep complete employment records. Where data were unavailable, we urged our respondents to make the best possible estimate. When facilities failed to respond after a few weeks, we began a follow-up of on-site visits. Numerous on-site visits were made to aid in the completion of the survey. Unfortunately, several large facilities reported that the complete information was not available, so estimates were made from other sources.

There are several other sources of hospital manpower data that supplemented and crosschecked our survey. The major sources were—

The Massachusetts Hospital Association's Annual Compensation Surveys for 1968, 1971, and 1973

The American Hospital Association's Annual Surveys for 1968, 1971, and 1973

The American Hospital Association's Nursing Survey for 1972

Unpublished data from the American Hospital Association

Through the data collected in the CMMS survey and supplemented by the sources referred to above, we were able to obtain the required information from all the hospitals in the survey area for each year. We were able to collect data concerning personnel and utilization rates from between 80 and 90 percent of the nursing and rest homes for the three study years. Data collection was difficult to obtain from ambulatory facilities because of their transitory nature. We did, however, obtain 1968 data from 80 percent of these facilities, 1971 data from 60 percent, and 1973 data from 78 percent of them (see table 1).

Our survey data refers to those facilities for which data was available directly or from alternate sources and does not reflect

Table 1. Facilities Included in Boston-Cambridge Survey

| Type of Provider | 1968 | | | 1971 | | | 1973 | | |
|---|---|---|---|---|---|---|---|---|---|
| | Total facilities | Facilities included in survey Number | Percent | Total facilities | Facilities included in survey Number | Percent | Total facilities | Facilities included in survey Number | Percent |
| Hospitals | 43 | 43 | 100.0 | 44 | 44 | 100.0 | 44 | 44 | 100.0 |
| Nursing or rest homes | 106 | 92 | 86.8 | 122 | 99 | 81.1 | 121 | 109 | 90.1 |
| Ambulatory facility | 55 | 44 | 80.0 | 80 | 48 | 60.0 | 96 | 75 | 78.0 |
| TOTAL | 204 | 179 | 87.7 | 246 | 191 | 77.6 | 261 | 228 | 87.4 |

**Source:** The Center for Medical Manpower Studies (CMMS), Northeastern University, Survey conducted in 1974 and 1975 of hospitals, nursing and rest homes, and ambulatory facilities in Boston and Cambridge.

the total of all employers of health personnel. Since we included the major employers and since our interest is in change over time, our failure to cover the universe should not substantially affect our findings.

## Utilization of Health Facilities

In addition to the manpower data, we needed utilization statistics from these facilities for the three years 1968, 1971, and 1973 in order to determine how the shifting patterns of the demand for health care had affected the staffing patterns of the facilities.

From hospitals we needed the following information:

1. number of licensed beds
2. number of inpatient days
3. number of inpatient admissions
4. average daily census
5. occupancy rate
6. number of ambulatory visits
7. types of medical facilities provided

From nursing and rest homes we needed the following:

1. number of beds
2. number of inpatient days
3. number of admissions
4. services available
5. number of Medicare days
6. number of public assistance days
7. number of private paying days

From ambulatory facilities we needed the following information:

1. number of visits, or
2. number of cases
3. services available

The sources of this information for Boston-Cambridge and the United States are as follows:

1. The 261 individual health providers in the study sample
2. The Commonwealth of Massachusetts Rate Setting Commission

    a. Nursing, Convalescent, Charitable Home for Aged and Rest Home Report (annual)

    b. The Commonwealth of Massachusetts Hospital Statement for Reimbursement (HCF-400 forms, annual)

3. The Annual Statistics gathered by the American Hospital Association

4. The Hospital Administrative Services Program (HAS) of the American Hospital Association

5. An unpublished print-out of hospital costs and facilities from the American Hospital Association

There was a considerable degree of overlap in the information collected from these sources, which proved helpful in crosschecking our overall results.

Analysis of the statistical information gathered has been made along the following lines:

1. the need for health manpower statistics

2. the allocation and utilization of health facilities during the period 1968 to 1973

3. the allocation and utilization of health manpower between 1968 and 1973

4. the significance of these statistics to the formation of health care policies by health providers and third party payers.

The occupations included in this study, along with functional descriptions of each, can be found in Appendix C. Many of these occupations were included because they represent large numbers of health workers. Others, such as nurse practitioner and physician's assistant, were included despite their relatively small number because they represent new trends in the training and utilization of health workers.

The list of occupations covers a wide range of professional training and educational backgrounds, from the most highly trained physician to the nurse's aide with no formal training requirements. In some occupations, such as laboratory technicians, electrocardiograph (EKG) and electroencephalograph (EEG) technicians, and inhalation therapists, one can find individuals with and without high levels of training and education.

# 3

## The Development of Hospitals in the United States

Although the health industry incorporates a wide range of activities, from the individual physician in private practice to the over-500-bed municipal hospital, the major employer of health personnel is the hospital. This study, however, will focus not only on hospitals but also on other health provider facilities, such as ambulatory centers and nursing and rest homes. Since approximately 85 percent of all health care workers are employed in hospitals, special emphasis must be given these facilities.

### The Flexner Report

Until the twentieth century hospitals in the United States functioned primarily for the poor, the aged, and the mentally ill, and relatively few restrictions were placed on the construction and growth of hospitals. As a result, the number of hospitals grew in a haphazard fashion through the first half of the twentieth century. Education and training of health personnel was also somewhat haphazard.

Of the estimated 3,500 physicians in the United States in 1775, only 400 held medical degrees.[1] Substantial changes were not made until well into the twentieth century. It was only after the publication in 1910 of what came to be known as the Flexner Report that serious attention was directed toward the regulation of medical schools and the general improvement of standards in hospitals.[2]

Late in the nineteenth century a conflict between hospitals and private practicing physicians developed over who would provide outpatient care for the poor. The physicians viewed the competition from outpatient clinics as a threat to their practices, and the physicians' views prevailed. As a result the development of outpatient departments by hospitals was neglected until after 1945, in spite of the obvious need for such services.

The Flexner Report not only resulted in an improved education for physicians and in better hospital facilities but also brought about a decrease in the physician/patient ratio. The country also experienced increased economic growth and prosperity. This combination of factors resulted in a lessening of competition between the physician and the hospital. The increase in cooperation between physicians and hospitals was strengthened as the physician became more dependent on well-equipped and well-staffed hospitals for the more sophisticated technology that had become available. Since 1945 full-time physicians (contractual physicians) have become more common, and by 1974 over 25 percent of the practicing physicians in the United States were contractual.

## Health Care Expenditures

Health care continues to be a rapid-growth industry in the United States, and the attention paid to the industry is easily understood when one considers the dollar value of activity in the area.

National health care expenditures accounted for 5.2 percent of the GNP in 1960, 5.9 percent in 1965, 7.5 percent in 1971, and 7.7 percent in 1973.[3] Hospital expenditures account for the largest single portion of these funds, 38.6 percent in 1973. In spite of the fact that consumers spend 56.3 percent of the total (government spends 38.9 percent and philanthropy 4.9 percent),[4] the widespread use of third-party payers partly shields the individual consumer from the direct costs of medical care.

Table 2 shows the growth of hospital expenditures relative to GNP between 1963 and 1973. It is noteworthy that in only two years of that ten-year period did the percentage rate of growth in the GNP exceed the percentage rate of growth in hospital expenditures. In most of the years in this period, hospital expenditures increased twice as much as the GNP. In 1971 and 1972 the hospital expenditure rate was only about 50 percent of the GNP growth rate, and by 1973 the rates were about equal. As is discussed later in this chapter, this slowdown may be linked to the increased attention devoted to this sector by certificate of need committees and third-party payers.

Since 1945 there has been an enormous increase in third-party medical coverage (health, medical, and hospital insurance). It has been estimated that by 1972 third parties met 90 percent of the hospital bill, 58 percent of the physician's bill, 13 percent of dental care and drug expenditures, and 60 percent of the remainder spent for all other services.[5] This increase in third-party coverage, accompanied by the quickening pace of medical technical equipopment, brought about a vast expansion of hospitals, services, and bed capacity in the United States. An indication of the magnitude of growth in the number of hospitals and in their utilization can be seen in table 3.

## Hospital Growth and Utilization

As calculated from table 3, between 1946 and 1973 the number of hospitals in the United States increased by 16.3 percent, and the number of hospital beds increased by 6.9 percent. However, the utilization pattern changed considerably; annual admissions more than doubled while the occupancy rate dropped by two percentage points. Although the average length of stay is not calculated for all U.S. hospitals, the 14 percent decrease in average length of stay for nonfederal short-term general and other special hospitals was indicative of the trend in most types of facilities. In

Table 2. Hospital Expenditures As a Percentage of Gross National Product, 1963-73

| | GNP | | Hospital Expenditures | | |
|---|---|---|---|---|---|
| Year | Amount (billions of dollars) | Increase from previous year (percent) | Amount (millions of dollars) | Increase from previous year (percent) | Percent of GNP |
| 1963 | 590.5 | 5.39 | 10,956 | 8.17 | 1.86 |
| 1964 | 632.4 | 7.10 | 12,031 | 9.81 | 1.90 |
| 1965 | 684.9 | 8.30 | 12,948 | 7.62 | 1.89 |
| 1966 | 749.9 | 9.49 | 14,198 | 9.65 | 1.89 |
| 1967 | 793.9 | 5.87 | 16,395 | 15.47 | 2.07 |
| 1968 | 864.2 | 8.86 | 19,061 | 16.26 | 2.07 |
| 1969 | 930.3 | 7.65 | 22,103 | 15.96 | 2.38 |
| 1970 | 977.1 | 5.03 | 25,556 | 15.62 | 2.62 |
| 1971 | 1,055.5 | 8.02 | 28,812 | 12.74 | 2.73 |
| 1972 | 1,155.2 | 9.45 | 32,667 | 13.38 | 2.83 |
| 1973 | 1,289.1 | 11.59 | 36,290 | 11.09 | 2.82 |

Source: American Hospital Association (AHA) Hospital Statistics, 1974, (Chicago: American Hospital Association, 1974), p. 5.

the same period the number of personnel employed in all hospitals in the United States increased by 234 percent, and the number of personnel per 100 census rose by over 200 percent. The total expenses for all hospitals showed a dramatic increase from $5.21 per patient day in 1946 to $83.67 per patient day in 1973.

The most marked increase during the 1946-73 period occurred in the nongovernmental short-term general and other special hospitals, which comprised 83 percent of all United States hospitals in 1973. The number of these hospitals increased by 32.6 percent, and the number of beds in these facilities nearly doubled.

Of the 7,123 registered hospitals in the United States in 1973, 5,891, or 82.7 percent, were in the category of nonfederal short-term general and other special hospitals. Such hospitals represent the most typical organizational structure; in 1973 they controlled 903,000 or 58.8 percent of the beds, 31,761,000 or 92.5 percent of the admissions, and 178,939,000 or 76.6 percent of the outpatient visits. The occupancy rate increased by 3.3 percent over this period, from 72.1 to 75.4, while the average length of stay decreased significantly from 9.1 to 7.8 days.

The number of personnel employed in these facilities also showed dramatic rates of growth, more than 300 percent from 1946 to 1973; during the last five years of this period, the number of workers employed increased by 68.3 percent. The number of personnel per 100 census more than doubled between 1946 and 1973, from 148 to 315.

As the health care industry has become more labor intensive, proportionately more workers have been required. The rapid growth in technology has required these workers to be more highly trained and therefore better paid. The total expenses per patient day increased more than tenfold; payroll expenses, which accounted for roughly half of all expenses, increased from $4.98 per patient day in 1946 to $63.86 per patient day in 1973.

Within the 1963-73 period the total number of admissions to all facilities increased by nearly 25 percent. Over the same years there has been a leveling off in hospital construction and addition of new beds. In fact, the total number of beds phased out in this decade exceeded the number of beds added. In this period the

Table 3. Trends in Hospital Utilization, by Classification, 1946, 1963, and 1973

| Classification | Year | Hospitals | Beds (thousands) | Inpatient | | | | | Outpatient visits (thousands) | Personnel | | |
|---|---|---|---|---|---|---|---|---|---|---|---|---|
| | | | | Admissions (thousands) | Average daily census (thousands) | Adjusted average daily census (thousands) | Occupancy (percent) | Average length of stay (days) | | Number (thousands) | Per 100 census | Per 100 adjusted census |
| United States, total | 1946 | 6,125 | 1,436 | 15,675 | 1,142 | | 79.5 | | 118,238 | 830 | 73 | |
| | 1963 | 7,138 | 1,702 | 27,502 | 1,430 | | 84.0 | | 233,555 | 1,840 | 129 | |
| | 1973 | 7,123 | 1,535 | 34,352 | 1,189 | | 77.5 | | | 2,769 | 233 | |
| Federal | 1946 | 404 | 236 | 1,593 | 166 | | 70.3 | | | 162 | 97 | |
| | 1963 | 446 | 176 | 1,598 | 152 | | 86.2 | | 29,473 | 206 | 135 | |
| | 1973 | 397 | 142 | 1,865 | 112 | | 79.0 | | 47,948 | 238 | 212 | |
| Nonfederal psychiatric | 1946 | 476 | 568 | 202 | 517 | | 91.0 | | 1,162 | 99 | 19 | |
| | 1963 | 499 | 715 | 435 | 657 | | 91.9 | | 4,611 | 261 | 40 | |
| | 1973 | 543 | 422 | 588 | 342 | | 81.1 | | | 303 | 88 | |
| Nonfederal tuberculosis and other respiratory diseases | 1946 | 412 | 75 | 85 | 55 | | 73.3 | | 632 | 36 | 66 | |
| | 1963 | 186 | 39 | 55 | 29 | | 73.0 | | 429 | 29 | 102 | |
| | 1973 | 63 | 10 | 26 | 6 | | 61.9 | | | 11 | 168 | |

| | 1946/1963/1973 | | | | | | | | | | |
|---|---|---|---|---|---|---|---|---|---|---|---|
| **Nonfederal long-term** General and other special | 1946 | 389 | 83 | 139 | 63 | 75.9 | | | | 28 | 45 | |
| | 1963 | 323 | 74 | 148 | 62 | 84.5 | | | 1,207 | 67 | 108 | 217 |
| | 1973 | 229 | 57 | 112 | 47 | 82.1 | | | 1,629 | 67 | 145 | 280 |
| **Nonfederal short-term general and other special, total** (totals of data in the following classifications): | 1946 | 4,444 | 471 | 13,655 | 341 | 72.1 | 9.1 | | | 505 | 148 | |
| | 1963 | 5,684 | 698 | 25,267 | 530 | 76.0 | 7.7 | 589 | 85,764 | 1,277 | 241 | |
| | 1973 | 5,891 | 903 | 31,761 | 681 | 75.4 | 7.8 | 768 | 178,939 | 2,149 | 315 | |
| **Nongovernmental not-for-profit short-term general and other special** | 1946 | 2,584 | 301 | 9,554 | 231 | 76.7 | 8.8 | | | 362 | 156 | |
| | 1963 | 3,394 | 486 | 18,120 | 377 | 77.7 | 7.6 | | 55,142 | 921 | 244 | |
| | 1973 | 3,320 | 629 | 22,488 | 489 | 77.8 | 7.9 | 545 | 120,273 | 1,535 | 314 | 282 |
| **For-profit short-term general and other special** | 1946 | 1,076 | 39 | 1,408 | 25 | 64.1 | 6.6 | | | 35 | 137 | |
| | 1963 | 896 | 44 | 1,832 | 30 | 68.0 | 6.1 | | 3,696 | 64 | 214 | |
| | 1973 | 757 | 63 | 2,334 | 43 | 68.3 | 6.7 | 47 | 7,593 | 117 | 272 | 249 |
| **State and local governmental short-term general and other special** | 1946 | 785 | 133 | 2,694 | 84 | 63.2 | 11.4 | | | 108 | 129 | |
| | 1963 | 1,394 | 168 | 5,315 | 123 | 73.0 | 8.5 | | 26,926 | 291 | 237 | |
| | 1973 | 1,814 | 211 | 6,939 | 149 | 70.6 | 7.8 | 176 | 51,072 | 497 | 333 | 283 |

**Source:** AHA *Hospital Statistics*, 1974, pp. 19 - 21.

total number of hospitals in the United States decreased slightly, while the total number of beds decreased by 9.8 percent. These declines took place in the categories of (a) federal and nonfederal psychiatric, (b) nonfederal tuberculosis, and (c) nonfederal long-term general and other special hospitals. The overall decrease in active staffed beds took place in noncommunity hospitals, which showed a 37.2 percent bed decrease. Community hospitals, defined as all nonfederal, short-term general hospitals whose facilities are available to the public, showed an increase of 29.4 percent. The decrease in noncommunity hospitals was primarily in psychiatric and tuberculosis hospitals.[6]

Overall utilization trends in United States hospitals are shown in table 4. Since 1946 the number of hospital beds per 1,000 population declined 25 percent, from a high of 10.1 beds per 1,000 population in 1946 to 7.3 beds per 1,000 population in 1973. During this entire period there was a continuous downward trend in the number of beds per 1,000 population and a continuous increase in the number of admissions per 1,000 population. In 1946 there were 110.4 admissions per 1,000 population; by 1973 the rate was 163.3 admissions, an increase of about 50 percent.

From this evidence one can infer that hospital facilities are more economically utilized now than before, and that the average length of stay per admission has also declined. Since the average daily census per 1,000 population has also steadily declined, one could tentatively conclude that the general health of the population may have improved.

One of the more significant changes during this period has been the substantial increase in hospital-based outpatient utilization. In 1963 the number of outpatient visits was 118.2 million, and by 1973 the number rose to 233.6 million. It is estimated that over 80 percent of this rise was due to increased utilization of the ambulatory facilities of nonfederal, short-term general and other special hospitals.

As noted above, the 1970s have seen reduced rates of growth in both hospitals and total bed capacity. One of the primary reasons has been the substantial increase in the cost of medical care. Some reasons for runaway health costs, particularly in-hospital costs, are more obvious than others. Increases in labor costs, the expansion of medical insurance programs, the relative geographic maldistribution of physicians, the implementation of new and more expensive medical techniques, and the relatively high profits of drug companies have all played a part in the spectacular price increases in medical care.

Although many categories of health workers still receive relatively low wages, there have been significant improvements. The gains can be attributed largely to unionization of some groups (especially the unskilled and semiskilled hospital workers) and to the increased economic activities of a growing number of professional organizations (especially among skilled and some semiskilled groups). Earnings of physicians always were relatively high, and they also have shown sharp increases. Physicians'

Table 4. Overall Trends in Hospital Utilization, United States,
Selected Years, 1946-73 ·

| | Hospital Beds | | Average Daily Census | | Admissions | |
| Year | Number (millions) | Per 1,000 population | Number (millions) | Per 1,000 population | Number (millions) | Per 1,000 population |
|---|---|---|---|---|---|---|
| 1946 | 1.436 | 10.1 | 1.142 | 8.0 | 15.675 | 110.4 |
| 1950 | 1.456 | 9.6 | 1.253 | 8.2 | 18.483 | 121.4 |
| 1955 | 1.604 | 9.6 | 1.363 | 8.2 | 21.073 | 127.0 |
| 1960 | 1.658 | 9.1 | 1.402 | 7.7 | 25.027 | 138.5 |
| 1961 | 1.670 | 9.1 | 1.393 | 7.6 | 25.474 | 138.7 |
| 1962 | 1.689 | 9.0 | 1.407 | 7.5 | 26.531 | 142.2 |
| 1963 | 1.702 | 9.0 | 1.430 | 7.5 | 27.502 | 145.3 |
| 1964 | 1.696 | 8.8 | 1.421 | 7.4 | 28.266 | 147.3 |
| 1965 | 1.704 | 8.7 | 1.403 | 7.2 | 28.812 | 148.3 |
| 1966 | 1.679 | 8.5 | 1.398 | 7.1 | 29.151 | 148.3 |
| 1967 | 1.671 | 8.4 | 1.380 | 6.9 | 29.361 | 147.7 |
| 1968 | 1.663 | 8.2 | 1.378 | 6.8 | 29.766 | 148.3 |
| 1969 | 1.650 | 8.1 | 1.346 | 6.6 | 30.729 | 151.6 |
| 1970 | 1.616 | 7.8 | 1.298 | 6.3 | 31.759 | 155.0 |
| 1971 | 1.556 | 7.5 | 1.237 | 5.9 | 32.664 | 157.7 |
| 1972 | 1.550 | 7.4 | 1.209 | 5.8 | 33.265 | 159.2 |
| 1973 | 1.535 | 7.3 | 1.189 | 5.6 | 34.352 | 163.3 |

Source: AHA *Hospital Statistics,* 1974, pp. 19-21; and U.S. Department of Commerce, Bureau of the Census, *Statistical Abstract of the United States,* 1974, (Washington: Government Printing Office, 1974), p. 5.

charges have increased more rapidly than the Consumer Price Index (CPI) in the United States because of the relatively inelastic demand for services.[7]

Increasingly over the last twenty years Americans have been covered by medical plans; at present well over 85 percent of all hospital bills are covered by third-party payers. At the same time a growing number of persons can now afford medical treatment, and they demand medical services. These factors would ordinarily lead to expansion of services and facilities, but the skyrocketing costs of health care in recent years brought about efforts to contain the expansion of these facilities.

## Certificate of Need Committees

Twenty-three of the fifty states have passed legislation to establish certificate of need committees. The prime responsibility of these committees is to monitor the pace in the growth of hospitals and bed capacity by evaluating the real need for new hospitals and additions to existing medical facilities. The approval of the certificate of need committees is required if any public (federal, state, or local) funds are to be used in the medical facility.

In Massachusetts the certificate of need law, passed in July 1972, required that construction of health facilities costing more than $100,000 be approved by the state. The law came in response to a belief that too much of the money available for health care was being spent on duplicative facilities in hospitals, diverting funds that might better be used for outpatient care and home care services.

A recent study completed in Massachusetts concluded that increasing the supply of beds produces a subsequent demand that fills them.[8] A review of certificate of need decisions conducted by the Massachusetts Department of Public Health found that, in the first eighteen months under the new law—

1. The overall number of beds in general hospitals seeking certificates of need dropped by 0.5 percent, from 5,272 to 5,247. These hospitals had asked to increase their supply of beds by 8 percent to 5,715.

2. The committee approved increases in the numbers of general hospital beds devoted to psychiatric care, rehabilitation and extended care, diabetes and alcoholism, though in smaller numbers than proposed by the applicant hospitals.

3. Within the subcategories of acute-care hospital beds, the study disclosed that hospitals applying for certificate of need had proposed a slight increase in the number of medical-surgical beds above the then-existing 4,053. The committee's actions resulted in reducing the number of such beds by 4 percent.

The mere fact that a state requires a certificate of need might diminish the requests by hospitals for unnecessary expansion. It is to be hoped that, as these committees apply their rules more strictly, fewer unneeded hospitals, beds, and other medical facilities will be constructed.

# 4

## The Utilization of Health Facilities

In this chapter we will focus on the changing utilization patterns of the various types of health providers during the 1968-73 study period. The discussion will begin with a description of all hospitals, followed by the utilization patterns of short-term, nonfederal hospitals. A similar presentation of the growth of nursing and rest home facilities describes the rapid development in this sector of the health care industry. Finally, we present data on ambulatory care facilities—including neighborhood health centers, clinics, and college infirmaries—which treat the so-called vertical patient.

### Hospital Trends in the United States—1968-73

Overall the total number of hospitals decreased slightly (0.2 percent), from 7,137 in 1968 to 7,123 in 1973 (see table 5). The number of hospital beds experienced a significant decrease of 7.7 percent. The total number of beds in federal hospitals decreased by 18 percent, those in nonfederal psychiatric facilities by 30 percent. Beds in nonfederal tuberculosis facilities showed a 46 percent decrease, and those in nonfederal long-term general decreased by 15 percent. Short-term nonfederal hospitals, representing over one-half of all beds in 1973, were the only group to show a net increase (12 percent).

The increase of 15.4 percent in admissions together with the decline in available beds failed to prevent the overall occupancy rate from falling from 82.9 (1968) to 77.5 (1973) percent. It is interesting to note that the occupancy rate declined in all subgroups, ranging from a 8.5 percentage point decline in nonfederal psychiatric facilities to 0.5 percentage point drop in nonfederal long-term general facilities. The mean average decline among all sub groups was greater than 4 percentage points.

The average daily census showed a reduction of more than 13 percent among all facilities. However, this statistic coupled with the increase of 15.4 percent in admissions indicates that the average length of stay among all facilities declined during the 1968-73 period.

Over the same five years the number of reported outpatient visits increased dramatically. The increase of almost 50 percent in

Table 5. Selected Utilization Measures, All U.S. Hospitals, 1968, 1971, and 1973

| Utilization Measure | 1968 | 1971 | 1973 | Percent Change 1968-1971 | 1971-1973 | 1968-1973 |
|---|---|---|---|---|---|---|
| Hospitals | 7,137 | 7,097 | 7,123 | −0.6 | 0.4 | −0.2 |
| Beds (thousands) | 1,663 | 1,556 | 1,535 | −6.4 | −1.4 | −7.7 |
| Average number beds per hospital | 233 | 219.2 | 215.5 | −6.0 | −1.7 | −7.5 |
| Admissions (thousands) | 29,766 | 32,664 | 34,352 | 9.7 | 5.2 | 15.4 |
| Average daily census (thousands) | 1,378 | 1,237 | 1,189 | −10.2 | −3.9 | −13.7 |
| Occupancy (percent) | 82.9 | 79.5 | 77.5 | −4.1 | −2.5 | −6.5 |
| Outpatient visits (thousands) | 156,139* | 199,725 | 233,555 | 27.9 | 16.9 | 49.6 |

Source: AHA *Hospital Statistics,* 1974, pp. 19-21.

*Based only on hospitals reporting outpatient visits.

outpatient utilization did not have a significant effect on the utilization of inpatient facilities. Rather, the increase in demand for outpatient services was brought about by the recognition that development of alternatives would be more appropriate and cost-effective to meet the increased demand for health services. These considerations may have been prompted to some degree by the increased use of hospital emergency rooms in place of a family physician, particularly in low-income areas of the inner city.

Our contention—that the accommodation of outpatient services did not seriously affect inpatient utilization—is supported in the next section, which deals with the group of short-term, nonfederal facilities.

## Short-Term Nonfederal Hospitals, United States and Boston-Cambridge, 1968-73

Short-term nonfederal hospitals represent 83 percent of all hospitals, employ 78 percent of all hospital personnel, and make 92 percent of all hospital admissions. They are more representative of the health care industry than any other group of hospitals, and the American Hospital Association provides more detailed statistics for this group than for any other. Tables 6 and 7 present the key utilization statistics for short-term nonfederal facilities in the United States and in the survey area for the years 1968, 1971, and 1973. The average length of stay in hospitals declined nationally from 8.4 days in 1968 to 7.8 days in 1973. In the Boston-Cambridge area the length of stay was considerably higher throughout the period; the figures were 11.6 in 1968 and 10.8 in 1971, and then rose to 11.3 in 1973. The occupancy rates for hospitals in the nation and in the Boston-Cambridge area were significantly different, and the changes over time were in different directions. The national rate was 78.2 percent in 1968 and declined slowly to 75.4 percent in 1973. The Boston-Cambridge rate was a bit higher in 1968 (81.0) and rose slowly to 82.8 in 1973.

The basic problem in comparing occupancy rates over time is that the base of the index (the number of beds) changes from year to year. An occupancy rate can drop drastically from one year to the next because of a sharp rise in the number of beds, with no change in any other factor. To avoid this problem, a utilization index was calculated by recomputing the occupancy rates with the number of beds held constant. Thus, using the number of beds in 1968 as the base, the occupancy rate was recalculated for the years 1971 and 1973, and the resulting figure was called the utilization

Table 6. Selected Utilization Measures, Short Term Nonfederal Hospitals
United States and Boston-Cambridge, 1968, 1971, and 1973[1]

| Utilization measure | 1968 United States | 1968 Boston-Cambridge | 1971 United States | 1971 Boston-Cambridge | 1973 United States | 1973 Boston-Cambridge |
|---|---|---|---|---|---|---|
| Hospitals | 5,820 | 29 | 5,843 | 29 | 5,891 | 30 |
| Beds | 806,000 | 7,529 | 884,000 | 7,382 | 903,000 | 7,526 |
| Average length of stay (days) | 8.4 | 11.6 | 7.9 | 10.8 | 7.8 | 11.3 |
| Outpatient visits (thousands) | 114,097 | 1,569 | 166,983 | 1,867 | 178,939 | 2,061 |
| Occupancy (percent) | 78.2 | 81.0 | 75.2 | 81.0 | 75.4 | 82.8 |
| Utilization index[2] | 78.2 | 81.0 | 82.5 | 79.4 | 84.5 | 82.6 |

Source: National figures taken from AHA, *Hospital Statistics,* annual; and *AHA Guide to the Health Care Field*, annual. Boston-Cambridge figures calculated from data published in *AHA Guide to the Health Care Field*, annual.

1. Before 1972 this category included hospital units of institutions, such as college and prison infirmaries, which are not available to the general public. These facilities were excluded from the category in 1972. In any comparisons between data for United States short-term nonfederal hospitals before 1972 and data for later years, one should note this exclusion of about 100 such facilities from 1972 on.

2. Occupancy rate adjusted according to number of beds in 1968 (see text).

index. For the nation as a whole the utilization index rose substantially from 78.2 in 1968 to 84.5 in 1973; in Boston-Cambridge the index rose only slightly, from 81.0 to 82.6.

The relative changes in the utilization of hospitals give an even clearer picture of how Boston-Cambridge hospitals compare with others. Over the five-year period from 1968 to 1973 the number of hospitals in the Boston-Cambridge area rose by 3.4 percent, but the number of beds declined by 0.04 percent; in the nation at the same time, the number of hospitals rose by a mere 1.2 percent while the number of beds increased by a sizable 12.0 percent.

Table 7. Changes in Utilization of Short-Term Nonfederal Hospitals,
United States and Boston-Cambridge, 1968-73[1]
(in percent)

| Utilization measure | 1968-71 | | 1971-73 | | 1968-73 | |
|---|---|---|---|---|---|---|
| | United States | Boston-Cambridge | United States | Boston-Cambridge | United States | Boston-Cambridge |
| Hospitals | 0.4 | 0.0 | 0.8 | 3.4 | 1.2 | 3.4 |
| Beds | 9.7 | −2.0 | 2.1 | 2.0 | 12.0 | 0.0 |
| Average length of stay (days) | −6.0 | −6.9 | −1.3 | 4.6 | −7.1 | −2.6 |
| Outpatient visits | 46.4 | 19.0 | 7.2 | 10.4 | 56.8 | 31.4 |
| Occupancy (percent) | −3.8 | 0.0 | 0.3 | 2.2 | −3.6 | 2.2 |
| Utilization Index[2] | 5.5 | −2.0 | 2.4 | 4.0 | 8.1 | 2.0 |

Source: Calculated from Table 6.

1. Before 1972 this category included hospital units of institutions, such as college and prison infirmaries, which are not available to the general public. These facilities were excluded from the category in 1972. In any comparisons between data for United States short-term nonfederal hospitals before 1972 and data for later years, one should note this exclusion of about 100 such facilities from 1972 on.

2. Occupancy rate adjusted according to number of beds in 1968 (see text).

While the occupancy rate and the utilization index both rose by approximately 2 percent over the five-year period in Boston-Cambridge hospitals, the rates diverged markedly for the various hospitals. For the nation, the occupancy rate actually dropped by 3.6 percent while the utilization index rose by 8.1 percent, a divergence due largely to the substantial increase in the number of hospital beds.

One other measure of hospital utilization is the number of outpatient visits, a hospital service that has shown substantial increases in recent years. Over the five-year period of our study, the number of outpatient visits showed a 31.4 percent increase in the Boston-Cambridge hospitals and a 56.8 percent increase nationally.

Of the twenty-two facilities in the Boston-Cambridge area for which occupancy rates are available for the entire five-year period, fourteen facilities showed a decrease in occupancy, having a mean average decline of 6.5 percent; eight facilities experienced an increase in occupancy with a mean rise of 5.8 percent. Significant also is the change in total bed capacity and change in the occupancy rate in individual hospitals. Six hospitals decreased bed capacity and nevertheless experienced a decline in occupancy. Six facilities increased their numbers of beds and their occupancy rates during the survey period. Five other hospitals that increased their total numbers of beds experienced a decline in occupancy. One municipal hospital cut back its bed capacity by more than 50 percent and still had an occupancy rate decline of nearly 6 percent. Of the four facilities that did not change their bed capacity, three showed significant losses and one experienced a slight gain in occupancy during the survey period. If the facilities that increased their bed capacity had been more sensitive to decreases in demand for inpatient services, their losses in occupancy could have been avoided by eliminating unneeded beds. It is just this lack of responsiveness in the health care system that has stimulated the current debate on the overcapacity of hospitals.

Nationally there was a significant decline in the number of small hospitals, with about a 30 percent decline in the number of beds in hospitals with a bed size of 6 to 24, and a 12 percent decline of beds in hospitals with a bed size of 25 to 49. The groupings of larger hospitals showed increases in the number of beds over the five-year period from 1968 to 1973 (see tables 8 and 9).

Since the survey area contained only twenty-nine facilities, the percentage changes in the number of beds by facility size often reflect the shifting in one facility. For example, in the Boston-Cambridge area there was a decrease of 27.9 percent in the number of beds in facilities with more than 500 beds and an accompanying increase of 111.1 percent in the number of beds in facilities with between 400 and 499 beds. This was accounted for by the shutdown of a number of beds at a municipal hospital.

Tables 8 and 9 present key utilization statistics for short-term nonfederal hospitals, by size, in the United States and in the survey area of Boston-Cambridge. In general, the data from the survey area demonstrates that facilities were better utilized in the Boston-Cambridge area than throughout the United States. To some extent this is true because of the specialized nature of some of the services offered by hospitals in the survey area; for the same reason the average length of stay in those hospitals were significantly longer than the national average in all size categories for the three survey years. The total number of outpatient visits increased in all categories in both the survey area and the United States as a whole. Moreover, the two largest facilities in the Boston-Cambridge area provided the largest percentage of total outpatient visits in the survey area—40 percent of all visits in 1968, 38 percent in 1971, and 37 percent in 1973.

## National Trends in Nursing and Rest Homes

The nursing and rest home industry had a tremendous growth spurt during the last decade, primarily as a result of the passage of the Medicare and Medicaid programs and also because of increasing numbers of older citizens, increased health insurance coverage, and improvements in medical technology. All of these factors contributed to an increase in demand for nursing care outside of hospitals, but it was the passage of the two new federal

Table 8. Utilization of Short-Term Nonfederal Hospitals, United States, by Size, 1968, 1971, and 1973

| Size (number of beds) | 1968 | | | | 1971 | | | | 1973 | | | |
|---|---|---|---|---|---|---|---|---|---|---|---|---|
| | Hospitals | Occupancy (percent) | Avg. Length of stay (days) | Outpatient Visits | Hospitals | Occupancy (percent) | Avg. length of stay (days) | Outpatient Visits | Hospitals | Occupancy (percent) | Avg. length of stay (days) | Outpatient Visits |
| 6-24 | 445 | 53.0 | 6.1 | 868,493 | 342 | 50.1 | 5.6 | 1,483,839 | 341 | 49.8 | 5.9 | 1,408,720 |
| 25-49 | 1,395 | 65.7 | 6.8 | 5,896,779 | 1,271 | 59.0 | 6.4 | 8,737,229 | 1,229 | 58.0 | 6.2 | 8,177,985 |
| 50-99 | 1,477 | 72.6 | 7.4 | 9,780,131 | 1,511 | 65.9 | 6.8 | 15,618,476 | 1,525 | 66.2 | 7.0 | 17,112,679 |
| 100-199 | 1,232 | 76.6 | 7.9 | 19,765,309 | 1,262 | 72.1 | 7.3 | 28,578,135 | 1,279 | 72.3 | 7.3 | 31,023,084 |
| 200-299 | 566 | 80.7 | 8.6 | 20,031,404 | 625 | 77.6 | 7.7 | 28,378,505 | 643 | 77.4 | 7.6 | 32,267,794 |
| 300-399 | 335 | 82.3 | 9.2 | 16,753,686 | 368 | 79.5 | 8.1 | 25,346,646 | 372 | 80.3 | 8.0 | 26,347,216 |
| 400-499 | 169 | 83.0 | 9.9 | 11,463,242 | 205 | 81.2 | 8.3 | 18,604,071 | 213 | 81.3 | 8.2 | 19,324,629 |
| 500 and over | 201 | 81.8 | 14.8 | 29,547,285 | 259 | 80.6 | 9.5 | 40,236,260 | 269 | 81.1 | 9.3 | 43,276,564 |
| Total | 5,820 | 78.2 | 8.4 | 114,097,329 | 5,843 | 75.2 | 7.9 | 166,983,161 | 5,891 | 75.4 | 7.8 | 178,938,671 |

Source: AHA *Hospital Statistics*, 1969, 1972, and 1974.

44

Table 9. Utilization of Short-Term, Nonfederal Hospitals, Boston-Cambridge, by size, 1968, 1971, and 1973

| Size (number of beds) | 1968 | | | | 1971 | | | | 1973 | | | |
|---|---|---|---|---|---|---|---|---|---|---|---|---|
| | Hospitals | Occupancy (percent) | Avg. length of stay (days) | Outpatient Visits | Hospitals | Occupancy (percent) | Avg. length of stay (days) | Outpatient Visits | Hospitals | Occupancy (percent) | Avg. length of stay (days) | Outpatient Visits |
| 6-24 | 0 | – | – | – | 0 | – | – | – | 0 | – | – | – |
| 25-49 | 1 | 70.2 | 10.5 | 0 | 2 | 66.7 | 12.6 | 6,348 | 2 | 67.9 | 9.6 | 7,400 |
| 50-99 | 5 | 80.1 | 12.0 | 10,781 | 5 | 77.3 | 11.9 | 10,784 | 5 | 70.2 | 11.2 | 13,026 |
| 100-199 | 10 | 66.4 | 11.1 | 225,393 | 9 | 76.8 | 11.3 | 277,013 | 9 | 76.1 | 11.9 | 289,729 |
| 200-299 | 3 | 73.0 | 12.3 | 90,190 | 2 | 77.7 | 8.9 | 42,490 | 3 | 74.3 | 10.2 | 108,558 |
| 300-399 | 7 | 87.8 | 11.6 | 536,601 | 8 | 82.2 | 9.9 | 751,938 | 7 | 82.5 | 11.3 | 694,553 |
| 400-499 | 1 | 80.0 | 9.8 | 75,023 | 1 | 69.5 | 9.0 | 71,318 | 2 | 86.7 | 11.4 | 192,534 |
| 500 and over | 2 | 81.0 | 11.8 | 629,436 | 2 | 83.6 | 12.0 | 707,143 | 2 | 94.4 | 10.2 | 755,541 |
| Total | 29 | 81.0 | 11.6 | 1,569,424 | 29 | 81.0 | 10.8 | 1,867,034 | 30 | 82.8 | 11.3 | 2,061,341 |

Source: AHA *Guide to the Health Care Field*, 1969, 1972, and 1974, and Massachusetts Rate Setting Commission, unpublished data.

45

health programs that gave the industry additional momentum. The 1965 amendments to the Social Security Act (Medicare) provided for up to 100 days of skilled nursing care in a certified facility for those aged 65 or over. The 1967 Medicaid program extended medical benefits to infirmed, disabled, and blind persons who are eligible for public assistance payments.

The intermediate care concept included in these programs was important in determining the structure of the industry. Intermediate care can be defined in a broad sense as less than skilled care and more than rest home care. It became apparent that there was a need for facilities that could provide long-term nursing care for those who need less than the care available in skilled nursing facilities.[1] The costs of individual states have been controlled somewhat under this provision because patients requiring less than skilled nursing care can be moved to a less expensive facility and remain under Medicare.

In the first five years of these federally funded programs the number of residents in such facilities increased dramatically. Between 1964 and 1969 there was a 47.1 percent increase in the number of residents in nursing and personal care homes in the United States, as the numbers rose from 554,000 to 815,100. In 1969 these 815,100 were residents in approximately 18,000 homes; nearly 89 percent of these residents were over the age of 65, and the median age for all residents was 81.[2] By 1973 the number of residents in these facilities was 1,098,500—an increase of nearly 35 percent over the figure for 1969.

The number of residents does not provide a complete picture of the activity of the industry, however, since it does not indicate the flow of persons into and out of such homes. In 1972, for example, 1,018,300 persons were admitted to nursing homes, an increase of nearly 8 percent over comparable 1967 statistics. Also in 1972, however, 984,600 residents were discharged from nursing homes, an increase of 13 percent over 1967.[3]

As shown in table 10, according to the National Center for Health Statistics, the total number of facilities providing nursing or personal care increased from 16,701 in 1963 to 22,004 in 1971, a increase of 31.8 percent. Of the four categories included, the most

Table 10. Nursing Care Homes and Related Facilities, with Total Bed Capacity, United States, 1963, 1969, and 1971*

| | FACILITIES | | | | | | BED CAPACITY | | | | | |
|---|---|---|---|---|---|---|---|---|---|---|---|---|
| | Number | | | Percent change | | | Number | | | Percent change | | |
| Classification | 1963 | 1969 | 1971 | 1963-1969 | 1969-1971 | 1963-1971 | 1963 | 1969 | 1971 | 1963-1969 | 1969-1971 | 1963-1971 |
| Nursing care | 8,128 | 11,484 | 12,871 | 41.3 | 12.1 | 58.4 | 319,224 | 704,217 | 917,707 | 120.6 | 30.3 | 187.5 |
| Personal care with nursing | 4,958 | 3,514 | 3,568 | -29.1 | 1.5 | -28.0 | 188,306 | 174,874 | 192,347 | -7.1 | 10.0 | 2.2 |
| Personal care without nursing | 2,927 | 3,792 | 5,369 | 29.6 | 41.6 | 83.4 | 48,962 | 63,532 | 88,317 | 29.8 | 39.0 | 80.4 |
| Domiciliary care | 688 | 120 | 196 | -82.6 | 63.3 | -28.5 | 12,068 | 1,253 | 3,227 | -89.6 | 157.5 | -73.3 |
| Total | 16,701 | 18,910 | 22,004 | 13.2 | 16.4 | 32.0 | 568,560 | 943,876 | 1,201,598 | 66.0 | 27.3 | 111.3 |

Source: U.:S. Department of Health, Education and Welfare, National Center for Health Statistics (NCHS) *Health Resources Statistics*, 1974 (Washington: Government Printing Office, 1974), p. 383.

*Facilities providing some form of nursing, personal, or domiciliary care are classified according to the primary or predominant service provided, as follows:

1. A *nursing care home* is defined as one in which 50 percent or more of the residents receive one or more nursing services and in which at least one registered nurse (RN) or licensed practical nurse (LPN) is employed thirty-five or more hours per week.

2. A *personal care home with nursing care* is defined as one in which either (a) some, but less than 50 percent, of the residents receive nursing care, or (b) more than 50 percent of the residents receive nursing care, but no RNs or LPNs are employed full time on the staff.

3. A *personal care home without nursing care* is defined as one which routinely provides no nursing service but three or more of the following personal services: rub or massage service; or assistance with bathing, dressing, correspondence, or shopping, with walking or getting about, or with eating.

4. A *domiciliary care home* is one which routinely provides less than three of the personal services specified above and no nursing service. This type of facility provides a sheltered environment primarily for persons who are able to care for themselves.

remarkable increase was in the number of personal care homes without nursing care, which increased by approximately 83 percent. The largest category, homes that provide nursing care, increased by 58.4 percent. The number of personal care homes with nursing declined 28.0 percent, and the number of domiciliary care homes dropped by 71.5 percent.

Although these survey years do not coincide exactly with our survey, the changes recorded between 1969 and 1971 are significant to our analysis. The total number of homes increased by 16.4 percent nationwide within the two-year period. Of all these facilities, homes that provided nursing care (more than half of all homes) increased by more than 12 percent, while personal care homes without nursing experienced a growth of 41.6 percent.

Nationally the number of beds in these facilities increased dramatically from 568,560 beds in 1963 to 1,201,598 in 1971, for a total change of 111.3 percent. Nursing care beds increased most dramatically, by 187.5 percent, while beds in personal care homes with nursing increased only slightly (2.2 percent) and those in personal care homes without nursing increased by 80.4 percent.[4]

Between 1969 and 1971 the number of beds in nursing care homes increased by 30.3 percent, and in personal care homes with nursing the increase was 10 percent. In the two non-nursing facility types the changes were more marked. In personal care homes without nursing the number of beds increased by nearly 40 percent within the two-year period; in homes providing domiciliary care the number of beds increased by more than 150 percent.

It is also interesting to note that the average size of these facilities increased by 57 percent between 1963 and 1971. The average number of beds in all facilities increased from 34.0 in 1963 to 54.6 in 1971. The facilities providing nursing care increased their average number of beds from 39.3 1963 to 71.3 in 1971, which is an 82 percent increase. Homes providing personal care with nursing increased their average bed capacity by 42 percent, from 38 beds to 54 beds. The total number of beds in those facilities providing only domiciliary care decreased by 73 percent. As of 1971, 78 percent of nursing and related homes—representing 67 percent of the beds—were privately owned and operated for profit.[5]

In interpreting these statistics it is worth noting that, although nursing homes are required to be licensed in each state, the standards and regulations are not uniform. Thus, the term *nursing home* encompasses facilities that provide skilled nursing care as well as those that offer little more than custodial care.

The number of residents of nursing and related homes in 1971 has been estimated at 1.1 million, approximately 5.2 percent of the population over age 65.[6] Of these, 77 percent are residents in nursing care homes, 16 percent in personal care homes with nursing, and 7 percent in personal care homes without nursing or in domiciliary care homes.

## Nursing and Rest Homes in Boston-Cambridge

Nursing homes are required to be licensed in each of the fifty states, but the standards, rules, and regulations describing levels of care vary from state to state. Massachusetts has a four-level classification, but detailed data before 1973 are not available except to distinguish between rest homes and all other levels of nursing facilities.

In the sample area of Boston and Cambridge the total number of nursing and rest home facilities increased 14.2 percent, from 106 in 1968 to 121 in 1973 (see table 11). In fact, a 15.1 percent increase occurred between 1968 and 1971, when for a short time there were 122 facilities. The total number of beds in these facilities increased by 27.5 percent over the five-year period.

There is no doubt that the implementation and wide acceptance of Medicare in this area proved to be a boost to the nursing home / rest home industry. In our sample twelve existing facilities expanded, and sixteen new facilities were opened. Of the sixteen new facilities that opened between 1968 and 1971, twelve were rest homes.

As shown in table 11, during the period of growth (1968-71) the occupancy rates in nursing and rest homes fell by 1.4 and 3.8 percent respectively. Within the next two years the occupancy rate in nursing homes rose significantly, to almost 100 percent of capacity. However, the rest homes did not fare as well. The group of rest homes in the survey area expanded too rapidly, and the occupancy rate fell by 13.8 percent between 1971 and 1973. In spite of some erratic patterns of development, the industry can be described as one with potential for additional growth. Much of the success in the nursing and rest home industry is a direct result of its proprietary nature. For-profit businesses generally react to changing demand more quickly than nonprofit organizations.

One of the reasons why the occupancy rate in these facilities is high is that there is no necessity to maintain empty beds for emergencies. As reported by the National Center for Health Statistics in the "1973-74 Nursing Home Survey," many of the more desirable facilities maintain waiting lists. There has been a steady increase in the number of nursing homes that maintain occupancy rates of over 80 percent, while the percentage reporting a rate of less than 70 percent has been reduced by half. In rest homes the opposite occurred. Over the survey period the occupancy rate in many of these facilities declined, so that in 1971 only 72.8 percent

Table 11. Utilization of Nursing and Rest Homes, Boston-Cambridge, 1968, 1971, and 1973

| Utilization measure | 1968 | 1971 | 1973 | Percent Change 1968-1971 | 1971-1973 | 1968-1973 |
|---|---|---|---|---|---|---|
| Facilities | 106.0 | 122.0 | 121.0 | 15.1 | −0.8 | 14.2 |
| Beds | 6200.0 | 7747.0 | 7905.0 | 25.0 | 2.0 | 27.5 |
| Occupancy (percent) | | | | | | |
| Nursing homes | 91.8 | 90.5 | 99.1 | −1.4 | 9.5 | 8.0 |
| Rest homes | 94.8 | 91.2 | 78.6 | −3.8 | −13.8 | −17.1 |
| Total | 94.1 | 90.3 | 96.1 | −4.0 | 6.4 | 2.1 |

Source: CMMS survey; and Massachusetts Rate Setting Commission, unpublished data.

reported occupancy rates of 80 percent or more, and 8.2 percent reported rates below 70 percent. This trend continued; by 1973 only 70.6 percent of rest homes in the sample reported occupancy rates of over 80 percent, whereas nearly 12 percent reported under 70 percent occupancy.


## Ambulatory Facilities in Boston-Cambridge

In spite of the predominance of hospital outpatient departments as providers of care to the "vertical patient," we will focus on the group of non-hospital-based ambulatory facilities, including neighborhood health centers, health maintenance organizations, and clinics.

Since this group represents the newest and most flexible type of health providers, data are difficult to acquire. In conducting the survey, it soon became obvious that the record keeping by these facilities was not always consistent. Moreover, since Massachusetts did not require ambulatory facilities to be licensed, the exact number of such facilities in operation is unknown. Many facilities relocate and reorganize several times over a short period, which contributes to the difficulty of determining their rate of growth and their impact on the health care system.

According to the results of our survey in the Boston-Cambridge area, the number of ambulatory facilities increased by nearly 75 percent between 1968 and 1973, a rate that far surpassed the rates of growth of any other type of health providers surveyed (see table 12).

The number of visits to the facilities increased by more than 50 percent between 1968 and 1973. This rise may be accounted for in part by the availability of several new large ambulatory facilities, including the Harvard Community Health Plan.

In addition to facilities reporting visits, approximately 10 to 12 percent of the ambulatory facilities tabulate utilization by counting numbers of cases, which can be defined as the number of individuals who utilized the facility in a given year. In spite of the obvious limitation in interpretation of these statistics, the average case load per facility reporting utilization in terms of the number of cases increased significantly in this period. Table 12 displays the growth pattern of the facilities that count the number of cases only. There has been an overall increase of 23.4 percent in the average case load per facility in the period 1968 to 1973.

Table 13 shows the distribution of ambulatory facilities in the Boston-Cambridge area by major type, for the years 1968, 1971, and 1973. As seen from this table, the remarkable growth in neighborhood health centers far outshadows the growth in any other facility type. The number of centers rose from seven to thirty-eight over a five-year period, an increase of 442 percent. The number of clinics showed an increase of 45 percent, and mental health centers increased by 23 percent. The overall increase of all ambulatory facilities was 74.5 percent over the five-year period. Moreover, as in the nursing and rest home category, the growth came largely between 1968 and 1971, after which the rate of increase fell off rapidly. One may note, however, that the number of facilities in each category is small, and that large percentage increases may give an exaggerated impression of growth.

The categories of care available within the ambulatory facilities in the survey area in 1973 are reported in table 14. General mental health services are offered by more than half the facilities; alcoholism treatment, a more specialized health service, is available in 22.0 percent of all facilities, and drug abuse treatment is available

Table 12. Utilization of Ambulatory Facilities, Boston-Cambridge, 1968, 1971, and 1973.

| | Year | | | Percent change | | |
|---|---|---|---|---|---|---|
| | | | | 1968- | 1971- | 1968- |
| Utilization measure | 1968 | 1971 | 1973 | 1971 | 1973 | 1973 |
| Facilities[1] | 55 | 80 | 96 | 45.5 | 20.0 | 74.5 |
| Visits | 1,317,289 | 1,992,782 | 1,999,600 | 51.3 | 0.3 | 51.8 |
| Average caseload[2] | 1,300 | 1,621 | 1,604 | 24.7 | −0.1 | 23.4 |

Source: CMMS survey.

1. Excluding outpatient departments of hospitals.
2. Total number of cases divided by number of facilities that reported utilization only in this way.

in 10.4 percent. The demand for mental health services has increased rapidly in the last few years, and the ambulatory setting has proved to be the least costly provider of this kind of care. Many patients who previously were unable to afford such services now avail themselves of them.

About one-half of all facilities surveyed offer such services as family planning, general medicine, obstetrics and gynecology, and pediatrics. In addition, because of their flexibility these facilities offer social services not traditionally available in a health care environment.

The outpatient departments of hospitals also serve an important role in providing health services similar to those of the ambulatory facilities. For a complete picture, both types of facilities should be combined. Table 15 shows the number of all outpatient visits provided by ambulatory facilities and hospitals in Boston-Cambridge for 1968, 1971, and 1973. Within the five-year period under study the total number of ambulatory visits to all providers increased by 40.7 percent. However, the 31.4 percent increase in visits provided by hospitals was surpassed by the 51.8 percent increase in the visits provided by ambulatory facilities.

The growth in outpatient visits to hospitals between 1968 and 1973 was 31.4 percent, showing an increase of nearly 20 percent

Table 13. Ambulatory Facilities, Boston-Cambridge, 1968, 1971 and 1973

| | Number | | | Percent change | | |
|---|---|---|---|---|---|---|
| Type of Facility | 1968 | 1971 | 1973 | 1968-1971 | 1971-1973 | 1968-1973 |
| Clinics | 11 | 12 | 16 | 9.1 | 33.3 | 45.4 |
| Neighborhood health center | 7 | 30 | 38 | 328.5 | 26.6 | 442.8 |
| Mental health center | 13 | 14 | 16 | 7.1 | 14.2 | 23.1 |
| College infirmary | 5 | 5 | 5 | – | – | – |
| Dental school or clinic | 7 | 7 | 7 | – | – | – |
| Other | 12 | 12 | 14 | – | 40.0 | 40.0 |
| TOTAL | 55 | 80 | 96 | 45.4 | 20.0 | 74.5 |

Source: CMMS survey.

between 1968 and 1971 and leveling off during the next two years. This contrasts sharply with the dramatic increase of 51.3 percent in outpatient visits to ambulatory facilities between 1968 and 1971 and the relative stabilization thereafter. Despite the fact that the number of visits provided by ambulatory facilities increased by over 50 percent in the five-year period, it is significant to note that in 1973 hospitals continued to provide slightly more than half of all outpatient visits.

## Neighborhood Health Centers

The concept of the neighborhood health center (NHC) arose out of the obvious need for primary health care providers in low-

Table 14. Categories of Health Care in Ambulatory Facilities,
Boston-Cambridge, 1973

| Category of Care | Percentage of Facilities Re- porting Service | Percentage Distribution of Services |
|---|---|---|
| Dental | 39.0 | 8.6 |
| Family planning | 48.0 | 10.6 |
| General medicine | 45.5 | 11.5 |
| Internal medicine, general | 13.0 | 2.0 |
| Mental health, general | 54.7 | 12.1 |
| Mental health, specialized | | |
|    Alcoholism | 22.0 | 4.9 |
|    Drug abuse | 10.4 | 2.3 |
|    Mental retardation | 6.4 | 1.4 |
|    Other | 13.0 | 2.8 |
| Obstetrics and gynecology | 50.0 | 11.1 |
| Ophthalmology/optometry | 26.0 | 5.5 |
| Pediatrics | 46.8 | 10.4 |
| Speech/hearing/physical therapy | 24.7 | 5.5 |
| Podiatry | 13.0 | 2.8 |
| Acupuncture | 1.3 | 0.2 |
| Nutrition | 32.5 | 7.2 |
| Other | 5.2 | 1.1 |
|    Total | n.a. | 100.0 |

Source: CMMS survey.

**Table 15. Utilization of Outpatient Facilities, Boston-Cambridge, 1968, 1971, and 1973**

| Outpatient facility | 1968 Visits | Distribution (percent) | 1971 Visits | Distribution (percent) | 1973 Visits | Distribution (percent) | Percent change 1968-71 | 1971-73 | 1968-73 |
|---|---|---|---|---|---|---|---|---|---|
| Hospital | 1,569,424 | 54.4 | 1,867,034 | 48.4 | 2,061,341 | 50.8 | 19.0 | 10.4 | 31.4 |
| Ambulatory facility | 1,317,289 | 45.6 | 1,992,782 | 51.6 | 1,999,600 | 49.2 | 51.3 | 0.3 | 51.8 |
| TOTAL | 2,886,713 | 100.0 | 3,859,816 | 100.0 | 4,060,941 | 100.0 | 33.7 | 5.2 | 40.7 |

Source: CMMS survey

55

income neighborhoods. Surveys of the emergency rooms of Boston City Hospital and the Massachusetts General Hospital[7] demonstrated that the majority of patients seen were not emergencies at all and that they generally had no private physician. In addition, surveys in several areas of the city noted the lack of primary care physicians in low-income urban areas.

The problem in the delivery of health care to the poor is not solely a matter of money. The purpose of Medicaid was to subsidize the poor so they could receive care from private practitioners. However, there were relatively few physicians in low-income neighborhoods, and the outpatient departments of hospitals were not adequate to provide primary care to these persons. The NHC was devised to fill the gap.

The neighborhood health centers generally provide five major services: adult medicine, pediatrics, family planning, maternity care, and mental health. Nonmedical services, such as nutrition, health education, and various social services, are also offered. In general, these services were not previously available in other ambulatory facilities.

Neighborhood health centers in Boston developed with no real effort at coordination among the various interest groups involved. There are several sources for funding of these facilities and because of this, each interest group (Model Cities, Office of Economic Opportunity, and permanent charities) located a facility in an area for its own reasons. As a result there are several competing facilities in close proximity, all providing comprehensive family care, while in other parts of the city such care is unavailable.

The northern section of Roxbury, for example, has a number of centers. Roxbury Comprehensive Community Health Center was funded in 1967; but before it opened its doors in 1969, another center opened, the Roxbury Medical and Dental Goup, and an existing well-baby clinic on Whittier Street was expanded. Model Cities opened a facility, the Mary Eliza Mahoney Center, nearby; the Black Panthers set up a free clinic, the Franklin Lynch People's Free Health Center. Within a limited geographic area, five facilities compete for clients.[8]

The city of Cambridge approached the problem by providing

care to its inner city residents in a unique fashion. It established seven clinics utilizing pediatric nurse practitioners (PNPs) to screen, diagnose, and treat pediatric patients. These clinics are located in neighborhood schools and provide easy access to those large population groups most in need of such services. The PNPs at these clinics provide primary and well-child care, thereby relieving the emergency room of The Cambridge Hospital. The results of this program have been significant in two ways. First, the program serves approximately 30 percent of the pediatric population of the city and 50 percent of the pediatric population in the five target areas in which health centers are located.[9] Second, the program supplied 18,000 patient visits in 1972, and at the same time the hospital's pediatric emergency room was relieved of much of its traffic for minor problems.

*University Infirmaries*

This study of ambulatory facilities includes the infirmaries of five major universities in the Boston-Cambridge area. The number of patient visits reported rose dramatically from 351,602 in 1968 to 441,837 in 1973, an increase of 25.7 percent. At the same time the student population was increasing by only 6 percent.

This increase in utilization reflects a developing sophistication of the college infirmary's growing variety of services, such as mental health and counseling centers and gynecological and family planning care. Students can now find these services on campus, rather than having to seek outside assistance. In addition, the services provided by the college infirmaries simply are less expensive than similar services off campus.

# 5

## Employment in the Health Care Industry

As one might predict, employment in the health care industry is closely related to the utilization of facilities in the industry. The previous chapter discussed the facilities of the industry and the remarkable growth in numbers and in utilization during the period from 1968 to 1973. We estimate that employment in the health care industry[1] rose nationally by 22 percent, although not all sectors within the industry showed the same proportionate employment increases. In this chapter we will relate the observed changes in utilization patterns of health facilities to the employment of health workers.

Because of the large number of different occupations in the industry and the substantial lack of uniformity of job titles among health facilities, we selected twenty-one health occupation titles that are widely used and represent a major segment of all health workers employed in the industry. Since the health care industry relies heavily on the services of part-time employees, employment figures used in this study are in terms of the full-time equivalent (FTE) rather than of the total number of individuals employed.

### The National Scene

Accurate national employment data on health care employees by occupation are not readily available. Annual employment estimates are made by the National Center for Health Statistics (NCHS), U.S. Department of Health, Education and Welfare, and they admittedly are estimates. Many groups and agencies in the health field, including the American Public Health Association, have expressed strong misgivings as to the accuracy of NCHS estimates. Occupational employment data are often furnished by self-serving groups, such as the professional organization representing the employees of an occupation, and clearly such data can be questioned. Nevertheless, the figures are the best available, and they are used in this study.

There have been significant additions to the health care team since the beginning of this century. At that time there were three active members: the physician, the nurse, and the nurse's aide. As the demand for health care increased, accompanied by numerous scientific and technological developments, many new occupations were created. By 1974 the number was estimated at over 450 individual health care occupations.[2] Despite the duplicate titles for some occupations, it is an impressive figure.

Tables 16 and 17 display national employment levels for the twenty-one occupations included in our survey. Because some of the estimates are not updated, some occupations show little growth while others show phenomenal rates of increase.

The number of interns, residents, and all other physicians increased at approximately the same rate as total employment, maintaining their representation at about 11 percent. As a whole the three nursing occupations (registered nurse, licensed practical nurse, and nurse's aide) constitute the single largest group, approximately 72 percent of total employment in the selected occupations. Over the five-year period from 1968 to 1973, the numbers of registered nurses experienced a growth of 20 percent, licensed practical nurses 33 percent, and nurse's aides 16 percent. From these figures it would appear that employers chose to utilize middle level LPNs instead of the higher rated RNs and the less skilled NAs. Technical occupations requiring formal education also experienced significant growth in this period. The number of medical technologists (MTs) more than doubled, physical therapists increased by 22 percent, and inhalation therapists increased

## Table 16. Levels of Employment, Selected Health Occupations, United States, 1968, 1971, and 1973

| Occupation | 1968 Number | 1968 Distribution (percent) | 1971 Number | 1971 Distribution (Percent) | 1973 Number | 1973 Distribution (percent) |
|---|---|---|---|---|---|---|
| Intern, resident | 23,800 | 0.96 | 24,799 | 0.87 | 28,211 | 0.93 |
| All other physicians | 251,200 | 10.10 | 297,201 | 10.43 | 305,189 | 10.03 |
| Nurse practitioner, pediatric nurse practitioner | n.a. | – | n.a. | – | n.a. | – |
| Physician's assistant | n.a. | – | 450 | 0.03 | 900 | 0.03 |
| Registered nurse | 680,000 | 27.34 | 748,000 | 26.26 | 815,000 | 26.79 |
| Licensed practical nurse | 345,000 | 13.87 | 427,000 | 15.00 | 459,000 | 15.09 |
| Nurse's Aide, orderly | 786,000 | 31.60 | 875,000 | 30.72 | 910,000 | 29.91 |
| Nurse anesthetist | n.a. | – | n.a. | – | n.a. | – |
| Pharmacist | 124,000 | 4.98 | 130,745 | 4.59 | 132,900 | 4.37 |
| Radiologic technician | 75,000 | 3.01 | 85,000 | 2.98 | 100,000 | 3.29 |
| Medical technologist (MT) | 43,000 | 1.73 | 78,000 | 2.74 | 90,300 | 2.97 |
| Medical technician (CLA) | 61,000 | 2.45 | 65,000 | 2.28 | 67,000 | 2.20 |
| OR technician | 19,000 | 0.76 | 23,400 | 0.82 | 23,400 | 0.77 |
| Physical therapist | 13,500 | 0.54 | 15,000 | 0.52 | 16,500 | 0.54 |
| Physical therapy assistant | 7,000 | 0.28 | 9,000 | 0.31 | 8,100 | 0.27 |
| Social worker (B.A.) | 1,500 | 0.06 | 3,500 | 0.12 | 4,300 | 0.14 |
| Social worker (M.S.W.) | 22,700 | 0.91 | 25,500 | 0.90 | 29,500 | 0.97 |
| Inhalation therapist | 8,000 | 0.32 | 10,000 | 0.35 | 12,000 | 0.39 |
| Speech therapist | 17,900 | 0.72 | 17,900 | 0.62 | 26,500 | 0.87 |
| EKG technician | 6,500 | 0.27 | 9,500 | 0.34 | 9,500 | 0.31 |
| EEG technician | 2,500 | 0.10 | 3,400 | 0.12 | 4,000 | 0.13 |
| TOTAL | 2,487,600 | 100.00 | 2,848,395 | 100.00 | 3,042,300 | 100.00 |

Source: NCHS, *Health Resources Statistics,* 1969, 1972-3, 1974

by 50 percent. The number of social workers (B.A.) nearly tripled over the five-year period.

The hundreds of allied health occupations range in skill and training requirements from the university graduate to those without a high school diploma who can be trained on the job within a few weeks to perform the functions of an occupation. There is no general agreement in the industry on the specific education and training requirements of each of the numerous occupations. For that matter, there often are wide differences among hiring institutions in the same geographic area with regard to hiring-in practices for the same occupation. It is not uncommon for a hospital to

**Table 17. Changes in Levels of Employment, Selected Health Occupations, United States, (in percent), 1968-73**

| Occupation | Percent change | | |
|---|---|---|---|
| | *1968-71* | *1971-73* | *1968-73* |
| Intern, resident | 4.2 | 13.8 | 18.5 |
| All other physicians | 18.3 | 2.7 | 21.5 |
| Nurse practitioner, pediatric nurse practitioner | n.a. | n.a. | n.a. |
| Physician's assistant | – | 100.0 | – |
| Registered nurse | 10.0 | 9.0 | 19.8 |
| Licensed practical nurse | 23.8 | 7.5 | 33.0 |
| Nurse's aide, orderly | 11.3 | 4.0 | 15.8 |
| Nurse anesthetist | n.a. | n.a. | n.a. |
| Pharmacist | 5.4 | 1.6 | 7.2 |
| Radiologic technician | 13.3 | 17.6 | 33.3 |
| Medical technologist (MT) | 81.4 | 15.8 | 110.0 |
| Medical technician (CLA) | 6.6 | 3.1 | 9.8 |
| OR technician | 23.2 | – | 23.2 |
| Physical therapist | 11.1 | 10.0 | 22.2 |
| Physical therapy assistant | 28.6 | −10.0 | 15.7 |
| Social worker (B.A.) | 133.3 | 22.9 | 186.7 |
| Social worker (M.S.W.) | 12.3 | 15.7 | 30.0 |
| Inhalation therapist | 25.0 | 20.0 | 50.0 |
| Speech therapist | – | 48.0 | 48.0 |
| EKG technician | 46.1 | – | 46.1 |
| EEG technician | 36.0 | 17.6 | 60.0 |
| TOTAL | 14.5 | 6.8 | 22.3 |

Source: Calculated from Table 16.

require a high school education for a nurse's aide, for example, if it is possible to hire persons with that qualification. At the same time, other hospitals in the same area may not require the high school diploma. Some health facilities are relatively inflexible in their hiring requirements, whereas others are sufficiently flexible to lower their education or training requirements when the labor market is very tight. There have been no studies to determine what the realistic education and training requirements should be for all the health occupations.

Table 18 shows twenty allied health occupations that could be considered possible entry-level jobs. We concede that many hospitals, administrators, and health personnel may not agree completely with this selection; but in our past research with a large cross-section of hospitals and other health facilities, we have seen these occupations filled by persons with a minimum of education and very little on-the-job training. There was little question about the level of their performance on the job. In general, it is our assumption that if it can be done in some hospitals, it can probably be done in most others.

Total employment in the health industry rose from 3.7 million in 1968 to 4.4 million in 1973, an increase of 20 percent. As seen in Table 18, over the same five-year period the number of employees in our listing of entry-level occupations rose from 1.4 million to 1.9 million, and in 1973 they represented about 42 percent of total health industry employment. If one excludes the figures for ambulance attendant because of the significant change in usage of the term and category and the figures in occupations for which data were not available in 1968, the rise in employment in the remaining occupations was 23.2 percent. Of this selected group of occupations, several experienced substantially large absolute and percentage increases: medical record technicians, laboratory technicians, dietetic technicians, nurse's aides, home health aides, social work aides, and respiratory therapists (inhalation therapists).

Institutional employment of allied health manpower can be divided into three principal categories: hospitals, ambulatory facilities, and nursing and rest homes. National estimates of the number of health workers employed by each type of provider are

Table 18. Levels of Employment in Potentially Entry-Level Occupations, 1968, 1971 and 1973

| Occupation | 1968 Number | 1968 Distribution (percent) | 1971 Number | 1971 Distribution (percent) | 1973 Number | 1973 Distribution (percent) |
|---|---|---|---|---|---|---|
| Clinical laboratory technician and assistant | 61,000 | 1.6 | 67,000 | 1.5 | 67,000 | 1.5 |
| Dental assistant | 95,000 | 2.6 | 114,000 | 2.5 | 116,000 | 2.6 |
| Dental laboratory technician | 27,000 | 0.7 | 31,150 | 0.7 | 32,000 | 0.7 |
| Dietetic technician | 6,000 | 0.2 | 7,000 | 0.2 | 23,000 | 0.5 |
| Medical library clerk | 6,000 | 0.2 | 4,100 | 0.1 | 4,100 | 0.1 |
| Record technician | 26,000 | 0.7 | 43,000 | 1.0 | 43,000 | 1.0 |
| Nurse's aide | 786,000 | 21.2 | 875,000 | 19.4 | 910,000 | 20.5 |
| Home health aide | 14,000 | 0.4 | 25,000 | 0.6 | 28,000 | 0.6 |
| Occupational therapy aide | 5,500 | 0.1 | 6,500 | 0.1 | 6,500 | 0.1 |
| Optometric assistant | n.a. | – | 5,000 | 0.1 | 5,000 | 0.1 |
| Optometric technician | n.a. | – | 1,000 | 0.02 | 1,000 | 0.02 |
| Physical therapy assistant | 8,000 | 0.2 | 9,000 | 0.2 | 8,100 | 0.2 |
| Radiologic technician | 100,000 | 2.7 | 100,000 | 2.2 | 100,000 | 2.2 |
| Respiratory therapist | 8,000 | 0.2 | 12,000 | 0.3 | 12,000 | 0.3 |
| Health office services | 275,000 | 7.4 | 300,000 | 6.7 | 300,000 | 6.7 |
| Social work aide | 1,500 | 0.04 | 4,300 | 0.1 | 4,300 | 0.1 |
| Ambulance attendant* | n.a. | – | 5,600 | 0.1 | 207,000 | 4.6 |
| Animal technician | n.a. | – | n.a. | – | 5,000 | 0.1 |
| Electrocardiograph technician | 7,000 | 0.2 | 9,500 | 0.2 | 9,500 | 0.2 |
| Electroencephalograph technician | 3,000 | 0.1 | 3,500 | 0.1 | 4,000 | 0.1 |
| Total Employees in Selected Occupations | 1,429,000 | 38.6 | 1,622,650 | 36.1 | 1,887,500 | 42.2 |
| Total Active Health Employees | 3,706,350 | 100.0 | 4,502,250 | 100.0 | 4,448,250 | 100.0 |

Source: NCHS, *Health Resources Statistics,* 1974, 1972-73, 1969.

*The figure in the 1971 column represents hospital employees in 1969. The 1973 figure covers all ambulance attendants, whether employed in hospitals or elsewhere.

not available. However, some indication of the changing nature of the industry and of health manpower employment can be seen from the indices of utilization of health facilities (see table 7).

## The Boston-Cambridge Survey

Employment in the twenty-one major occupations of the health care industry in Boston-Cambridge rose from 19,774.0 in 1968 to 24,721.5 in 1973 (FTE), an increase of 25.2 percent (see tables 19 and 20). Over the same five-year period employment in these twenty-one occupations in the nation as a whole rose by 22.3 percent. The basic differences between the United States and the Boston-Cambridge data in the distribution of personnel involved interns and residents, licensed practical nurses, and nurse's aides. There was no uniform pattern of increase over the five-year period between the data for the nation and for Boston-Cambridge.

Over the five-year period studied, occupational groups representing large proportions of total employment showed substantial employment gains. Interns and residents showed a 17.5 percent gain; all other physicians a 35.0 percent gain; registered nurses were up by 26.7 percent; and nurse's aides and orderlies were up by 14.6 percent. The only major classification that showed a relatively small employment increase was licensed practical nurse, which rose by only 2.8 percent. Other occupations that represented substantial numbers were medical technologists and medical technicians, and they showed employment increases of 50.1 percent and 44.6 percent respectively.

In 1968 the interns, residents, and other physicians represented 19.4 percent of the health care employment in the survey area, and five years later they represented 19.6 percent. The nursing group of occupations (RN, LPN, and NA) was the major employment group; it represented 65.8 percent of the industry's employment in 1968 and dropped slightly to 61.8 percent in 1973. In calculations where the focus is on allied health employment, interns, residents, and other physicians are omitted. If this were done here, the nursing groups would have represented 81.6 percent of the total employment in 1968 and 76.8 percent in 1973.

Table 19.  Levels of Employment, Selected Health Occupations,
Boston-Cambridge, 1968, 1971 and 1973

| | 1968 | | 1971 | | 1973 | |
|---|---|---|---|---|---|---|
| Occupation | Num-ber (FTE)[1] | Distri-bution (percent) | Num-ber (FTE)[1] | Distri-bution (percent) | Num-ber (FTE)[1] | Distri-bution (percent) |
| Intern, resident | 1,973.0 | 10.0 | 2,207.0 | 9.4 | 2,318.0 | 9.4 |
| All other physicians | 1,853.5 | 9.4 | 2,301.5 | 9.8 | 2,502.5 | 10.2 |
| Nurse practitioner, pediatric nurse practitioner | 10.0 | 0.05 | 33.5 | 0.1 | 60.0 | 0.2 |
| Physician's assistant | 4.0 | 0.02 | 10.0 | 0.04 | 12.5 | 0.05 |
| Registered nurse | 5,702.5 | 28.9 | 6,893.0 | 29.4 | 7,222.5 | 29.3 |
| Licensed prac-tical nurse | 2,250.5 | 11.4 | 2,202.5 | 9.4 | 2,312.5 | 9.4 |
| Nurse's aide, orderly | 5,043.0 | 25.5 | 6,137.0 | 26.1 | 5,677.5 | 23.1 |
| Nurse anesthetist | 66.0 | 0.3 | 67.5 | 0.3 | 80.0 | 0.3 |
| Pharmacist | 137.0 | 0.7 | 147.5 | 0.6 | 164.0 | 0.7 |
| Radiologic technician | 171.5 | 0.8 | 474.5 | 2.0 | 528.0 | 2.1 |
| Medical tech-nologist (MT) | 539.0 | 2.7 | 575.0 | 2.4 | 809.0 | 3.3 |
| Medical tech-nician (CLA) | 746.0 | 3.7 | 893.0 | 3.8 | 1,078.5 | 4.4 |
| OR technician | 123.5 | 0.6 | 146.0 | 0.6 | 197.0 | 0.8 |
| Physical therapist | 190.0 | 0.9 | 238.5 | 1.0 | 265.0 | 1.1 |
| Physical ther-apy assistant | 55.5 | 0.3 | 70.5 | 0.3 | 91.0 | 0.4 |
| Social worker (B.A.) | 120.5 | 0.6 | 123.5 | 0.5 | 253.5 | 1.0 |
| Social worker (M.S.W.) | 478.0 | 2.4 | 588.0 | 2.5 | 596.5 | 2.4 |
| Inhalation therapist | 139.5 | 0.7 | 196.5 | 0.8 | 270.5 | 1.1 |
| Speech therapist | 29.5 | 0.1 | 39.5 | 0.2 | 51.0 | 0.2 |
| EKG technician | 82.5 | 0.4 | 100.5 | 0.4 | 94.5 | 0.4 |
| EEG technician | 29.0 | 0.1 | 30.0 | 0.1 | 41.0 | 0.2 |
| TOTAL | 19,744.0 | 99.57[2] | 23,475.0 | 99.74[2] | 24,628.0 | 100.2[2] |

Source: CMMS Survey.

1. FTE – full-time equivalent.
2. Totals may not add to 100 percent because of rounding.

The changing nature of the types of health industry employers in a large sample of institutional health providers in Boston and Cambridge can be seen in table 21. Over 200 health facilities are represented in this table for 1973, including 100 percent of all hospitals, 90 percent of all nursing and rest homes, and 78 percent of all ambulatory facilities.

During the 1968-73 period the number of health workers employed in Boston-Cambridge hospitals increased by 25.4 percent; hospitals maintained approximately 80 percent of total health facilities employment. Nursing and rest homes over the same period showed a decrease of 1.7 percent in the number of health

Table 20. Changes in Levels of Employment, Selected Health
Occupations, Boston-Cambridge, 1968-73

| Occupation | Percent change | | |
| | 1968-71 | 1971-73 | 1968-73 |
|---|---|---|---|
| Intern, resident | 11.2 | 5.7 | 17.5 |
| All other physicians | 24.1 | 8.8 | 35.0 |
| Nurse practitioner, pediatric | | | |
| nurse practitioner | 235.0 | 88.1 | 530.0 |
| Physician's assistant | 150.0 | 25.0 | 212.5 |
| Registered nurse | 20.9 | 4.8 | 26.7 |
| Licensed practical nurse | 2.1 | 5.0 | 2.8 |
| Nurse's aide, orderly | 21.7 | −7.5 | 12.6 |
| Nurse anesthetist | 2.3 | 18.5 | 21.2 |
| Pharmacist | 7.7 | 11.2 | 19.7 |
| Radiologic technician | 176.7 | 11.3 | 207.9 |
| Medical technologist (MT) | 6.6 | 40.8 | 50.1 |
| Medical technician(CLA) | 19.7 | 20.8 | 44.6 |
| OR technician | 18.2 | 34.9 | 59.5 |
| Physical therapist | 25.5 | 11.3 | 39.7 |
| Physical therapy assistant | 25.2 | 31.7 | 64.9 |
| Social worker (B.A.) | 2.5 | 105.3 | 110.4 |
| Social worker (M.S.W.) | 23.0 | 1.4 | 24.7 |
| Inhalation therapist | 40.9 | 37.7 | 93.5 |
| Speech therapist | 33.9 | 13.9 | 52.5 |
| EKG technician | 21.8 | −6.0 | 14.5 |
| EEG technician | 3.4 | 36.7 | 41.4 |
| TOTAL | 18.8 | 5.4 | 25.2 |

Source: CMMS survey.

personnel employed. Employment in these homes in 1973 represented only 12.1 percent of total health employment in the area.
Ambulatory facilities showed the most impressive percentage
increase in employment; the numbers almost doubled over the
five-year period. Total health manpower employment during the
1968-73 period for all health facilities in the sample area increased
by 24.7 percent.

As shown in table 21, in 1973 hospitals employed about four of
every five health care workers in Boston-Cambridge; nursing
homes employed about 12 percent and ambulatory facilities about
8 percent. The percentage change in employment over the five-
year period varied significantly among the three basic types of
facilities. The utilization of the hospital facilities from 1968 to
1973 showed a decrease of beds of 0.04 percent, a rise in the occupancy rate of 1.8 percent, and a rise of 31.3 percent in the number
of outpatient visits. With these changes in the utilization of hospitals there was an increase in health care employment. Over the
five-year period studied, hospital employment increased to a
greater extent than did the utilization of hospital facilities.

The vast majority of hospital employees are related to inpatient
facilities, not to outpatient services. The utilization of inpatient
facilities, as measured by the occupancy rate, rose by only 1.8 percent while employment rose by over 25 percent. The conclusion
one may draw from such a relationship is that there has been a
substantial rise in the medical services performed per patient,
requiring considerably more health manpower to serve the same
number of patients. This increase in demand resulted partly from
biomedical research, partly from new technologies and equipment, and partly from new concepts of maximum care. (See tables
22 and 23 for a distribution of employment by selected health
occupations in hospitals in Boston-Cambridge.)

While the number of ambulatory facilities in Boston-Cambridge increased by 74.5 percent over the five-year period from
1968 to 1973 and the number of visits to these facilities rose by 51
percent, employment in these facilities showed a dramatic rise of
97.9 percent. Again, the increase in employment outstripped the
increases in facilities and utilization. The only possible explana-

Table 21. Distribution of Health Workers, by Type of Employer, Boston-Cambridge, 1968, 1971, and 1973

| Employer | 1968 Number (FTE)[1] | 1968 Distribution (percent) | 1971 Number (FTE)[1] | 1971 Distribution (percent) | 1973 Number (FTE)[1] | 1973 Distribution (percent) | Percent change 1968-71 | Percent change 1971-73 | Percent change 1968-73 |
|---|---|---|---|---|---|---|---|---|---|
| Hospital | 15,760.5 | 79.8 | 18,633.5 | 79.4 | 19,759.0 | 80.2 | 18.2 | 6.0 | 25.4 |
| Nursing or rest home | 3,027.0 | 15.4 | 3,245.0 | 13.8 | 2,977.0 | 12.1 | 7.2 | -8.3 | -1.7 |
| Ambulatory facility | 956.5 | 4.8 | 1,596.5 | 6.8 | 1,892.0 | 7.7 | 66.9 | 18.5 | 97.8 |
| TOTAL | 19,744.0 | 100.0 | 23,475.0 | 100.0 | 24,628.0 | 100.0 | 18.9 | 4.9 | 24.7 |

Source: CMMS survey.

1. FTE – full-time equivalent.

69

tion for this rather large increase in employment is the increase in available services at ambulatory centers.

The positive relationship between facilities and utilization on the one hand, and employment on the other, did not hold for nursing and rest homes. Over the five-year period studied the number of such facilities rose by 15 percent, the number of beds increased by 27.6 percent, and the occupancy index (adjusted for the increase in number of beds) rose by 30.3 percent. Despite this marked increase in the utilization of nursing and rest homes, employment in these facilities actually declined by 1.7 percent during the last two years of the period, 1972 and 1973 (see tables 24 and 25). This may be explained at least in part by the fact that, while occupancy rates of nursing homes rose by 8.0 percent over the five-year period, rest homes showed an occupancy rate decline of 17.1 percent. Rest homes apparently overexpanded during this period, causing the marked drop in occupancy. Another possible explanation of the employment decline is that the required level of service in these facilities, as measured by the proportion of qualified employees to patients has declined.

As indicated above, the nursing group of occupations (RN, LPN, and NA) represents about 65 percent of the industry's employment. Table 26 shows the percentage distribution of each of the three major nursing occupations by type of health care provider. Hospitals are the major employer of these occupations; they employ about 87 percent of all registered nurses, but approximately 70 percent of the LPNs and only 64 percent of the nurse's aides. In 1973 nursing homes employed only about 5 percent of the RNs, 28 percent of the LPNs, and 33 percent of the NAs. The major change in distribution occurred between 1968 and 1971, when nursing homes decreased their share of registered nurses from 8.0 percent to 5.7 percent and ambulatory facilities increased their share of LPNs from 61.0 percent to 69.4 percent and nursing homes decreased their share from 36.9 percent to 27.7 percent.

Tables 22 through 25 and tables 27 and 28 show the employment of the twenty-one major categories of health occupations in 1968, 1971, and 1973, for each of the three types of health care employers (hospitals, nursing and rest homes, and ambulatory

Table 22. Levels of Employment, Selected Health Occupations,
Hospitals, Boston-Cambridge, 1968, 1971, and 1973

| Occupation | 1968 Number (FTE)[1] | 1968 Distribution (percent) | 1971 Number (FTE)[1] | 1971 Distribution (percent) | 1973 Number (FTE)[1] | 1973 Distribution (percent) |
|---|---|---|---|---|---|---|
| Intern, resident | 1,891.0 | 12.00 | 2,093.0 | 11.23 | 2,151.5 | 10.89 |
| All other physicians | 1,615.5 | 10.25 | 1,919.0 | 10.30 | 2,073.5 | 10.49 |
| Nurse practitioner, pediatric nurse practitioner | 10.0 | 0.07 | 31.5 | 0.17 | 43.5 | 0.22 |
| Physician's assistant | 4.0 | 0.03 | 10.0 | 0.05 | 11.0 | 0.06 |
| Registered nurse | 5,072.0 | 32.18 | 5,997.5 | 32.19 | 6,336.5 | 32.07 |
| Licensed practical nurse | 1,373.0 | 8.71 | 1,529.0 | 8.21 | 1,607.5 | 8.14 |
| Nurse's aide, orderly | 3,212.0 | 20.38 | 3,825.5 | 20.53 | 3,655.5 | 18.50 |
| Nurse anesthetist | 66.0 | 0.41 | 67.5 | 0.36 | 80.0 | 0.40 |
| Pharmacist | 129.5 | 0.82 | 141.5 | 0.76 | 159.0 | 0.80 |
| Radiologic technician | 158.5 | 1.02 | 449.5 | 2.41 | 491.0 | 2.48 |
| Medical technologist (MT) | 497.0 | 3.15 | 521.5 | 2.80 | 738.5 | 3.74 |
| Medical technician (CLA) | 711.0 | 4.51 | 839.0 | 4.50 | 982.5 | 4.97 |
| OR technician | 123.5 | 0.78 | 146.0 | 0.79 | 197.0 | 1.00 |
| Physical therapist | 172.0 | 1.10 | 215.0 | 1.15 | 243.0 | 1.24 |
| Physical therapy assistant | 51.0 | 0.32 | 64.0 | 0.34 | 75.5 | 0.38 |
| Social worker (B.A.) | 78.0 | 0.50 | 78.5 | 0.42 | 112.0 | 0.56 |
| Social Worker (M.S.W.) | 318.0 | 2.02 | 343.0 | 1.84 | 358.5 | 1.81 |
| Inhalation therapist | 139.5 | 0.88 | 196.5 | 1.05 | 267.5 | 1.35 |
| Speech therapist | 27.5 | 0.17 | 37.5 | 0.20 | 42.0 | 0.22 |
| EKG technician | 82.5 | 0.52 | 98.5 | 0.53 | 92.5 | 0.47 |
| EEG technician | 29.0 | 0.18 | 30.0 | 0.17 | 41.0 | 0.21 |
| TOTAL | 15,760.5 | 100.00 | 18,633.5 | 100.00 | 19,759.0 | 100.00 |

Source: CMMS survey.

1. FTE – full-time equivalent

facilities). In hospitals the largest percentage increases were for nurse practitioner (335 percent), physician's assistant (175 percent), radiologic technician (210 percent), and inhalation therapist (91.8 percent); the absolute numbers involved in the first two occupations listed, however, were very small. The six occupations with the largest employment (intern and resident, all other physicians, registered nurse, licensed practical nurse, nurse's aide, and radiologic technician) showed increases ranging from 13.8 percent to 39.0 percent. Two unskilled hiring-in occupations, nurse's aide and physical therapy assistant, showed relatively modest increases over the five-year period.

Table 23. Changes in Levels of Employment, Selected Health Occupations
Hospitals, Boston-Cambridge, 1968-73

| | | Percent change | |
| Occupation | 1968-71 | 1971-73 | 1968-73 |
| --- | --- | --- | --- |
| Intern, resident | 10.7 | 2.8 | 13.8 |
| All other physicians | 18.8 | 8.1 | 28.4 |
| Nurse practitioner, pediatric nurse practitioner | 215.0 | 38.1 | 335.0 |
| Physician's assistant | 150.0 | 10.0 | 175.0 |
| Registered nurse | 18.2 | 5.7 | 24.9 |
| Licensed practical nurse | 11.4 | 5.1 | 17.0 |
| Nurse's aide, orderly | 19.1 | −4.4 | 13.8 |
| Nurse anesthetist | 2.3 | 18.5 | 21.2 |
| Pharmacist | 9.3 | 12.4 | 22.8 |
| Radiologic technician | 183.6 | 9.2 | 209.8 |
| Medical technologist (MT) | 4.9 | 41.6 | 48.6 |
| Medical technician (CLA) | 18.0 | 17.1 | 38.2 |
| OR technician | 18.2 | 34.9 | 59.5 |
| Physical therapist | 25.0 | 13.0 | 41.3 |
| Physical therapy assistant | 25.5 | 18.0 | 48.0 |
| Social worker (B.A.) | 0.6 | 42.7 | 43.6 |
| Social worker (M.S.W.) | 7.9 | 4.5 | 12.7 |
| Inhalation therapist | 40.9 | 36.1 | 91.8 |
| Speech therapist | 36.4 | 12.0 | 52.7 |
| EKG technician | 19.4 | −6.1 | 12.1 |
| EEG technician | 3.4 | 36.7 | 41.4 |
| TOTAL | 18.2 | 6.0 | 25.4 |

Source: CMMS survey.

Table 24. Levels of Employment, Selected Health Occupations, Nursing
and Rest Homes, Boston-Cambridge, 1968, 1971, and 1973

| Occupation | 1968 Number (FTE)[1] | 1968 Distribution (percent) | 1971 Number (FTE)[1] | 1971 Distribution (percent) | 1973 Number (FTE)[1] | 1973 Distribution (percent) |
|---|---|---|---|---|---|---|
| Intern, resident | – | – | – | – | – | – |
| All other physicians | – | – | – | – | 8.5 | 0.3 |
| Nurse practitioner, pediatric nurse practitioner | – | – | – | – | – | – |
| Physician's assistant | – | – | – | – | – | – |
| Registered nurse | 406.0 | 13.4 | 393.0 | 12.1 | 360.0 | 12.1 |
| Licensed practical nurse | 830.0 | 27.4 | 611.5 | 18.8 | 655.0 | 22.0 |
| Nurse's aide, orderly | 1,791.0 | 59.2 | 2,240.5 | 69.1 | 1,904.0 | 64.0 |
| Nurse anesthetist | – | – | – | – | – | – |
| Pharmacist | – | – | – | – | – | – |
| Radiologic technician | – | – | – | – | – | – |
| Medical technologist (MT) | – | – | – | – | – | – |
| Medical technician (CLA) | – | – | – | – | – | – |
| OR technician | – | – | – | – | – | – |
| Physical therapist | – | – | – | – | 6.5 | 0.2 |
| Physical therapy assistant | – | – | – | – | 10.5 | 0.4 |
| Social worker (B.A.) | – | – | – | – | 14.5 | 0.5 |
| Social worker (M.S.W.) | – | – | – | – | 12.0 | 0.4 |
| Inhalation therapist | – | – | – | – | – | – |
| Speech therapist | – | – | – | – | 6.0 | 0.2 |
| EKG technician | – | – | – | – | – | – |
| EEG technician | – | – | – | – | – | – |
| TOTAL | 3,027.0 | 100.0 | 3,245.0 | 100.0 | 2,977.0 | 100.1[2] |

Source: CMMS survey.

1. FTE – full-time equivalent.
2. Totals may not equal 100 percent because of rounding.

As shown in tables 24 and 25, nursing and rest homes employ personnel in a very limited number of health care occupations, principally the three nursing occupations: registered nurse, licensed practical nurse, and nurse's aide. In 1968 these nursing occupations represented nearly 100 percent of employment in these facilities, the nurse's aide representing 60 percent of the total. By 1973 a small number of workers in physical therapy and in social work were employed in such facilities, and these occupa-

Table 25. Changes in Levels of Employment, Selected Health Occupations, Nursing and Rest Homes, Boston-Cambridge, 1968-73

| Occupation | Percent change | | |
| | 1968-71 | 1971-73 | 1968-73 |
| --- | --- | --- | --- |
| Intern, resident | – | – | – |
| All other physicians* | – | – | – |
| Nurse practitioner, pediatric nurse practitioner | – | – | – |
| Physician's assistant | – | – | – |
| Registered nurse | −3.2 | −8.4 | −11.3 |
| Licensed practical nurse | −26.3 | 7.1 | −21.1 |
| Nurse's aide, orderly | 25.1 | −15.0 | 6.3 |
| Nurse anesthetist | – | – | – |
| Pharmacist | – | – | – |
| Radiologic technician | – | – | – |
| Medical technologist (MT) | – | – | – |
| Medical technician (CLA) | – | – | – |
| OR technician | – | – | – |
| Physical therapist* | – | – | – |
| Physical therapy assistant* | – | – | – |
| Social worker (B.A.)* | – | – | – |
| Social worker (M.S.W.)* | – | – | – |
| Inhalation therapist | – | – | – |
| Speech therapist* | – | – | – |
| EKG technician | – | – | – |
| EEG technician | – | – | – |
| TOTAL | 7.2 | −8.3 | −1.7 |

Source: CMMS survey.

*The facilities did employ personnel in these categories by 1973. See Table 24.

tions represented 1.7 percent of the total employment. In that year nurse's aides represented 64 percent of total employment in these facilities.

Over the five-year period studied, employment in nursing and rest homes declined by 1.7 percent, as a result of sharp drops in the number of registered nurses and licensed practical nurses employed. The former showed a drop of 11 percent and the latter 21 percent. Nurse's aides showed a rise of 6 percent. This shift in the utilization of nursing occupations indicates a tendency in nursing and rest homes to employ the less-skilled employees as a substitute for those with higher skills. Pressures for such a shift are caused by higher salaries as well as the relative shortage of registered nurses. In addition, administrators of nursing homes quickly realized that nurse's aides can readily perform a substantial portion of the functions normally charged to licensed practical nurses and even registered nurses.

In the ambulatory facilities the major occupational categories were physician, registered nurse, nurse's aide, and social worker. In 1973, all physicians represented 31.0 percent of employment in ambulatory facilities; registered nurses represented 27.8 percent; nurse's aides 2.6 percent; social workers (B.A.) 6.7 percent; and social workers (M.S.W.) 11.9 percent. Over the five-year period from 1968 to 1973, employment of registered nurses showed a 134 percent increase, nurse's aides 195 percent, social workers (B.A.) almost 200 percent, and social workers (M.S.W.) 41 percent. Medical technicians, though not a major occupation in the ambulatory facilities, have grown in importance over the five years; their numbers increased by 174 percent, and by 1973 they represented 5.1 percent of total employment in these facilities (see tables 27 and 28).

Our sample of ambulatory facilities included the infirmaries of five major universities in the Boston-Cambridge area. These are substantially different from other ambulatory facilities, and they employ a different distribution of health care occupations (see tables 29 and 30). Physicians and registered nurses together represented 70.1 percent of total employment in 1973. Dentists, dental hygienists, and dental assistants, none of them found in the other health care facilities surveyed, represented 13.0 percent of employment. Total employment of health care personnel rose by 19.2 percent in university infirmaries—a rate considerably less than the employment increase in other ambulatory centers, since the latter includes many facilities that did not exist in 1968.

Table 26. Distribution of Nursing Workers, by Type of Employer,
Boston-Cambridge, 1968, 1971 and 1973 (in percent)

| Occupation | Type of Employer | | | |
| | Hospital | Nursing home | Ambula-tory facilitiy | Total* |
|---|---|---|---|---|
| Registered nurse | | | | |
| 1968 | 88.0 | 8.0 | 4.0 | 100.0 |
| 1971 | 87.0 | 5.7 | 7.2 | 99.9 |
| 1973 | 87.7 | 5.0 | 7.3 | 100.0 |
| Licensed practical nurse | | | | |
| 1968 | 61.0 | 36.9 | 2.1 | 100.0 |
| 1971 | 69.4 | 27.7 | 2.8 | 99.9 |
| 1973 | 69.5 | 28.3 | 2.1 | 99.9 |
| Nurse's aide | | | | |
| 1968 | 63.7 | 35.5 | 0.8 | 100.0 |
| 1971 | 62.3 | 36.5 | 1.1 | 99.9 |
| 1973 | 65.0 | 32.9 | 2.0 | 99.9 |

Source: CMMS survey.

*Totals may not add to 100 percent because of rounding.

Table 27. Levels of Employment, Selected Health Occupations,
Ambulatory Facilities, Boston-Cambridge,
1968, 1971, and 1973

| | 1968 | | 1971 | | 1973 | |
|---|---|---|---|---|---|---|
| Occupation | Number (FTE)[1] | Distribution (percent) | Number (FTE)[1] | Distribution (percent) | Number (FTE)[1] | Distribution (percent) |
| Intern, resident | 82.0 | 8.6 | 114.0 | 7.1 | 166.5 | 8.8 |
| All other physicians | 238.0 | 24.9 | 382.5 | 24.0 | 420.5 | 22.2 |
| Nurse practitioner, pediatric nurse practitioner | – | – | 2.0 | 0.1 | 19.5 | 1.0 |
| Physician's assistant | – | – | – | – | 1.5 | 0.1 |
| Registered nurse | 224.5 | 23.4 | 502.5 | 31.5 | 526.0 | 27.8 |
| Licensed practical nurse | 47.5 | 5.0 | 62.0 | 3.9 | 50.0 | 2.6 |
| Nurse's aide, orderly | 40.0 | 4.2 | 71.0 | 4.4 | 118.0 | 6.2 |
| Nurse anesthetist | – | – | – | – | – | – |
| Pharmacist | 7.5 | 0.8 | 6.0 | 0.4 | 5.0 | 0.3 |
| Radiologic technician | 13.0 | 1.6 | 25.0 | 1.6 | 37.0 | 2.0 |
| Medical technologist (MT) | 42.0 | 4.4 | 53.5 | 3.4 | 70.5 | 3.7 |
| Medical technician (CLA) | 35.0 | 3.7 | 54.0 | 3.4 | 96.0 | 5.1 |
| OR technician | – | – | – | – | – | – |
| Physical therapist | 18.0 | 2.0 | 23.5 | 1.5 | 15.5 | 0.8 |
| Physical therapy assistant | 4.5 | 0.5 | 6.5 | 0.4 | 5.0 | 0.3 |
| Social worker (B.A.) | 42.5 | 4.4 | 45.0 | 2.8 | 127.0 | 6.7 |
| Social worker (M.S.W.) | 160.0 | 16.7 | 245.0 | 15.3 | 226.0 | 11.9 |
| Inhalation therapist | – | – | – | – | 3.0 | 0.2 |
| Speech therapist | 2.0 | 0.2 | 2.0 | 0.1 | 3.0 | 0.2 |
| EKG technician | – | – | 2.0 | 0.1 | 2.0 | 0.1 |
| EEG technician | – | – | – | – | – | – |
| TOTAL | 956.5 | 100.4[2] | 1,596.5 | 100.0 | 1,892.0 | 100.0[2] |

Source: CMMS survey.

1. FTE – full-time equivalent.
2. Totals may not add to 100 percent because of rounding.

**Table 28. Changes in Levels of Employment, Selected Health Occupations Ambulatory Facilities, Boston-Cambridge, 1968-73**

| Occupation | Percent change | | |
|---|---|---|---|
| | 1968-71 | 1971-73 | 1968-73 |
| Intern, resident | 39.0 | 46.1 | 103.0 |
| All other physicians | 60.7 | 9.9 | 76.6 |
| Nurse practitioner, pediatric nurse practitioner | – | 875.0 | – |
| Physician's assistant* | – | – | – |
| Registered nurse | 123.8 | 4.7 | 134.3 |
| Licensed practical nurse | 30.6 | 19.3 | 5.3 |
| Nurse's aide, orderly | 77.5 | 66.2 | 195.0 |
| Nurse anesthetist | – | – | – |
| Pharmacist | –20.0 | –16.6 | –33.3 |
| Radiologic technician | 92.3 | 48.0 | 184.6 |
| Medical technologist (MT) | 27.4 | 31.8 | 67.9 |
| Medical technician (CLA) | 54.3 | 77.7 | 174.3 |
| OR technician | – | – | – |
| Physical therapist | 30.6 | –34.0 | –13.9 |
| Physical therapy assistant | 44.4 | –23.1 | 11.1 |
| Social worker (B.A.) | 5.9 | 182.2 | 198.8 |
| Social worker (M.S.W.) | 53.1 | –7.8 | 41.2 |
| Inhalation therapist* | – | – | – |
| Speech therapist | – | 50.0 | 50.0 |
| EKG technician* | – | – | – |
| EEG technician | – | – | – |
| TOTAL | 66.9 | 18.5 | 97.8 |

Source: CMMS survey.

*The facilities did employ personnel in these categories by 1973, some by 1971. See table 27.

Table 29. Levels of Employment, Selected Health Occupations,
College Infirmaries, Boston-Cambridge, 1968, 1971 and 1973

| | 1968 | | 1971 | | 1973 | |
| Occupation | Number (FTE)[1] | Distribution (percent) | Number (FTE)[1] | Distribution (percent) | Number (FTE)[1] | Distribution (percent) |
|---|---|---|---|---|---|---|
| Intern, resident | 91.6 | 40.5 | 92.0 | 37.2 | 97.5 | 36.2 |
| All other physicians | 15.5 | 6.8 | 18.5 | 7.5 | 19.0 | 7.0 |
| Registered nurse | 61.5 | 27.2 | 72.1 | 29.1 | 72.6 | 26.9 |
| Licensed practical nurse | 4.0 | 1.7 | 4.0 | 1.6 | 5.0 | 1.9 |
| Nurse's aide, orderly | 8.0 | 3.5 | 8.0 | 3.2 | 12.0 | 4.5 |
| Pharmacist | – | – | – | – | 0.5 | 0.2 |
| Radiologic technician | 4.5 | 2.0 | 8.0 | 3.2 | 8.0 | 3.0 |
| Medical technologist (MT) | 6.0 | 2.6 | 6.5 | 2.6 | 6.5 | 2.4 |
| Medical technician (CLA) | 4.0 | 1.8 | 4.5 | 1.8 | 4.5 | 1.7 |
| Physical therapist | 1.0 | 0.4 | 2.0 | 0.8 | 2.0 | 0.7 |
| Physical therapy assistant | 3.0 | 1.3 | 4.0 | 1.6 | 3.0 | 1.1 |
| Social worker (B.A.) | – | – | – | – | 1.0 | 0.4 |
| Social worker (M.S.W.) | 1.0 | 0.4 | 2.0 | 0.8 | 2.0 | 0.7 |
| EKG technician | – | – | 1.0 | 0.4 | 1.0 | 0.4 |
| Dentist | 19.0 | 8.4 | 16.0 | 6.5 | 24.0 | 8.9 |
| Dental hygienist | 4.0 | 1.8 | 4.0 | 1.6 | 4.0 | 1.5 |
| Dental assistant | 3.0 | 1.3 | 5.0 | 2.0 | 7.0 | 2.6 |
| TOTAL | 226.1 | 99.7[2] | 247.6 | 99.9[2] | 269.6 | 100.1[2] |

Source: CMMS survey.

1. FTE – full-time equivalent.
2. Totals may not add to 100 percent because of rounding.

Table 30. Changes in Levels of Employment, Selected Health Occupations
College Infirmaries, Boston-Cambridge, 1968-73

| | Percent change | | |
|---|---|---|---|
| Occupation | 1968-71 | 1971-73 | 1968-73 |
| Intern, resident | 0.4 | 6.0 | 6.4 |
| All other physicians | 19.4 | 2.7 | 22.6 |
| Registered nurse | 17.2 | 0.7 | 18.0 |
| Licensed practical nurse | – | 25.0 | 25.0 |
| Nurse's aide, orderly | – | 50.0 | 50.0 |
| Pharmacist* | – | – | – |
| Radiologic technician | 77.8 | – | 77.8 |
| Medical technologist (MT) | 8.3 | – | 8.3 |
| Medicial technician (CLA) | 12.5 | – | 12.5 |
| Physical therapist | 100.0 | – | 100.0 |
| Physical therapy assistant | 33.3 | –25.0 | – |
| Social worker (B.A.)* | – | – | – |
| Social worker (M.S.W.) | 100.0 | – | 100.0 |
| EKG technician* | – | – | – |
| Dentist | –15.8 | 50.0 | 26.3 |
| Dental Hygienist | – | – | – |
| Dental assistant | 66.7 | 40.0 | 133.3 |
| TOTAL | 9.5 | 8.8 | 19.2 |

Source: CMMS survey.

*The facilities did employ personnel in these categories by 1973, some
by 1971. See table 29.

# 6

## Some International Comparisons

A comparison of industries across national borders may present a picture in which some countries suffer by comparison. Nations may differ significantly in terms of laws, institutions, customs, and age structures. A composite picture of an industry in one country may vary significantly from that in others, although the difference in real terms may not be great. Health care is a concern of all nations, and international comparisons have been made for many years, if for no other reason but to motivate a worldwide increase and improvement in the health services offered. Some comparisons are presented here in order to place the United States health care scene against a similar setting in a number of other countries.

Two trends relating to health and health manpower seem to transcend the international borders of West European countries and the United States. First, in most Organization for Economic and Community Development (OECD) nations, employment in the health area represents a significant and growing element of the total labor force (see table 31). The health care industry usually ranks as one of the five largest fields of employment, and in many OECD countries approximately 3 to 5 percent of the labor force finds employment in this area. As shown in table 31, from the early 1960s to the late 1960s a number of the OECD countries had

81

Table 31. Percentages of Total Labor Force Engaged in Health Care
Industry, Selected OECD Member Countries,
Selected Years, 1960-70

| | | | Health Care Industry* | |
| Country | Year | Total Labor Force | Number of Workers | Percentage of labor force |
|---|---|---|---|---|
| Australia | 1961 | 4,225,096 | 134,453 | 3.2 |
| | 1966 | 4,856,455 | 190,672 | 3.9 |
| Canada | 1961 | 8,471,830 | 307,515 | 1.8 |
| | 1970 | 8,374,000 | 502,282 | 6.0 |
| Denmark | 1960 | 2,007,639 | 76,981 | 3.8 |
| | 1965 | 2,198,628 | 94,407 | 4.3 |
| France | 1962 | 18,956,380 | 536,160 | 2.8 |
| | 1968 | 20,002,240 | 730,660 | 3.7 |
| Greece | 1961 | 3,638,601 | 38,708 | 1.1 |
| | 1971 | 3,283,880 | 40,680 | 1.2 |
| Ireland, (Republic of) | 1961 | 1,052,539 | 30,331 | 2.9 |
| | 1966 | 1,065,987 | 33,576 | 3.1 |
| Japan | 1960 | 43,690,500 | 647,266 | 1.5 |
| | 1971 | 50,630,000 | 961,000 | 1.9 |
| New Zealand | 1961 | 895,363 | 37,237 | 4.2 |
| | 1966 | 1,026,039 | 44,608 | 4.3 |
| Sweden | 1960 | 3,244,084 | 119,391 | 3.7 |
| | 1970 | 3,412,668 | 210,407 | 6.2 |
| United Kingdom | 1960 | 25,072,000 | 774,000 | 3.1 |
| | 1970 | 25,675,000 | 1,037,000 | 4.0 |
| United States | 1960 | 72,142,000 | 2,642,300 | 3.7 |
| | 1970 | 85,903,000 | 4,246,187 | 4.9 |

Source: Organization for Economic and Community Development,
*New Directions in Education for Changing Health Care
System*, (Paris: OECD, 1975), p. 32.

*All persons employed in the health industry, not only in health care
occupations.

substantial increases in health manpower, in each case greater than the rise in the total labor force.

A second trend that transcends international borders is the increasing specialization found in all health care systems. In the United States, as previously discussed, the number of health care occupations over the last fifty years has increased from three to well over 400. Similar trends can be documented in most OECD countries.

As shown in table 32, there is considerable variation in health indices among the nations listed. Only Germany and Italy have infant mortality rates higher than the rate in the United States, and the rate ranges from 11.5 per 1,000 live births in the Netherlands to 27.0 in Italy. An important measure of a nation's concern with health care is the health budget as a percent of gross domestic product (GDP). Again there is a significant variation; the percentage ranges from a low of 3.4 percent in Belgium to a high of 7.7 in the United States. Theoretically this index could measure the amount or quality of health services actually delivered, but in practice it fails to do so. There appears to be no consistent pattern among nations in the relation between the health budget index and the indices that present some measure of health service.

Table 33 presents data for the same nations on the number of health service personnel in selected occupations. The population per physician ranged from a low of 544 in Italy to a high of 960 in Ireland. Three of the nations listed had ratios lower than the United States. Italy's low figure may indicate quantity, but other health indices surely show that there need not be a close relationship between quantity and quality. The variation in the numbers employed in the selected occupations would seem to indicate that no single structure of health occupations is accepted worldwide. It would also seem to indicate that nations have different patterns of utilization of health care personnel and that certain occupations in one country are substituted for other occupations in other countries.

## Table 32. Health Indices, Selected Industrialized Countries

| Country | 1972 Infant mortality rate per 1,000 live births | Average life expectancy | 1971-72 Health budget percent of GDP | Total beds | Hospital Utilization | | | |
|---|---|---|---|---|---|---|---|---|
| | | | | | Population per bed | Admissions per 10,000 population | Average length of stay | 1970 Occupancy rate |
| Belgium | 18.1 | 70.0 (1963-66) | 3.4 | 80,392 | 120 | 1,071.1 (1970) | 14.2 | 86.9 |
| Denmark | 13.5 | M: 70.7 F: 75.6 (1968-69) | 4.2 | 47,440 | 100 | 1,520.2 | 13.1 | 87.8 |
| France: | 16.0 | M: 68.8 F: 76.1 (1970) | 8.0 | 539,700 | 100 | 719.6[1] | 17.8[1] | 77.5[1] |
| Germany | 22.8 | M: 67.2 F: 73.4 (1968-70) | n.a. | 683,254 | 90 | 1,439.1 | 18.3 | 88.5 |
| Ireland | 17.8 | M: 68.6 F: 72.8 (1966) | 3.9 | 37,084 | 80 | n.a. | n.a. | n.a. |
| Italy[2] | 27.0 | M: 68.5 F: 74.6 (1970) | 5.7[3] | 568,513 | 90 | 1,492.1 | 13.8 | 77.5 |
| Luxembourg | 14.0 | M: 66.0 F: 73.0 (1960-65) | n.a. | 3,910 | 90 | 1,263.6 | 14.7 | 81.5 |
| Netherlands | 11.5 | M: 71.0 F: 76.4 (1966-70) | n.a. | 156,555 | 80 | 967.1[4] | 18.5[4] | 89.0[4] |

| | | | | | | | | |
|---|---|---|---|---|---|---|---|---|
| England and Wales | 17.3 | M: 68.8 F: 75.2 (1970) | 3.8 | 445,387 | 110 | 1,087.8 | n.a. | 82.2 |
| United States[5] | 18.5 | M: 67.4 F: 75.2 (1972) | 7.7 | 1,550,000 | 130 | 1,611.2 | 8.9 | 78.0 |

**Sources:** Except as otherwise noted, all data are from World Health Organization, *Health Services in Europe* (Copenhagen: WHO, 1975). Additional data and verification are from United Nations, *Statistical Yearbook*, 1972 (New York: UN, 1973); and World Health Organization, *World Health Statistics Report*, 26 (Copenhagen: WHO, 1975). Most figures are for 1970, although some are for 1969 and 1971.

1. Public hospitals only.
2. All personnel estimates for Italy from United Nations, *Statistical Yearbook*, 1974, p. 784.
3. Estimated 1970 from OECD national accounts for member countries, *New Directions in Education for Changing Health Care System* (Paris: OECD, 1975), p. 31.
4. General hospitals only.
5. Calculations for United States are for 1972 and from American Hospital Association, *Hospital Statistics*, 1975. (Chicago: AHA, 1975).

Table 33. Health Manpower, Selected Industrialized Countries

| Country | Physicians Number | Population per physician | Midwife | Nurse | Nurse's Aide | Physio-therapist | Medical technician |
|---|---|---|---|---|---|---|---|
| Belgium | 15,500 (1972) | 630 | 3,333 | n.a. | n.a. | n.a. | n.a. |
| Denmark | 7,000 (1970) | 700 | 580 | 26,000[1] | 11,620 | 2,340 | n.a. |
| France | 71,000 (1973) | 721 | 9,000 | 150,000 | 150,000 | 20,500 | n.a. |
| Germany | 114,771 (1972) | 572 | 6,505 | 185,792 | 2,748 | 19,856 | 15,934[3] |
| Ireland | 3,011 | 960 | —[4] | 16,067[4] | n.a. | n.a.[5] | n.a.[5] |
| Italy | 99,341 (1971)[6] | 544 | 18,828 | 127,399 | —[7] | n.a. | 156,055[7] |
| Luxembourg | 368 (1971) | 924 | 90 | 667[8] | —[8] | n.a. | n.a. |
| Netherlands | 17,381 (1972) | 760 | 883 | 50,114[9] | n.a. | 1,195 | 6,971[10] |
| England and Wales | 70,122 | 771 | 19,258 | 180,679 | 99,92 | 7,687 | 7,045 |
| United States | 322,000 (1971)[11] | 641 | 4,950 | 175,000[12] | 875,000 | 15,000 | 145,000[13] |

86

**Source:** Except as otherwise noted, all data are from World Health Organization, *Health Services in Europe* (Copenhagen: WHO, 1975). Additional data and verification are from United Nations, *Statistical Yearbook, 1972* (New York, UN, 1973), and World Health Organization, *World Health Statistics Report*, 26 (Copenhagen: WHO, 1975). Most figures are for 1970, although some are for 1969 and 1971.

1. One-third are part-time.
2. One-quarter are part-time.
3. Surgery and laboratory assistants.
4. Midwives and nurses are combined.
5. These occupations are not subject to statutory registration in Ireland.
6. Includes dentists, who must first earn an M.D. before specializing in dentistry.
7. Nursing aides, laboratory assistants, and radiologic technicians are combined under Medical Technician; from *Annuario Di Statistiche Sanitarie*, 1971-72.
8. Nurses and nursing assistants are combined.
9. Includes public health nurses and student nurses.
10. Includes radiologic and laboratory technicians.
11. Data for the United States from *Health Resources Statistics, 1972-73*, Table 1, pp. 8-11.
12. Registered nurses and licensed practical nurses.
13. Laboratory technologists and technicians.

# 7

## Summary and Conclusions

To some extent this study was undertaken because of the concern that hospital occupancy rates were no longer rising, and in some cases were actually falling. Under such conditions the nation's expanding education and training programs for health care occupations could create a substantial surplus of allied health personnel in a stable (or perhaps declining) labor market. Various aspects of the health care industry are discussed in this report. An analysis is made of the utilization of health care facilities, but the principal focus is health care manpower—specifically on what has happened to employment in the industry during the five-year period from 1968 to 1973. If it could be shown that health care employment rose during this period despite the apparent decline in the utilization of facilities, it would be evidence that other factors in the industry are creating a growth in demand for allied health personnel. Our survey covered the health care facilities and employment in the Boston-Cambridge area over the five-year period.

### Health Care Facilities and Their Utilization

The total number of hospitals in the United States did not change markedly over the decade 1963 to 1973, dropping only 0.2

89

percent, but the total number of beds declined by 9.8 percent during the same period. However, there has been a considerable shift away from long-term federal and psychiatric facilities, accompanied by an expansion of short-term nonfederal hospitals. Excluding federal and long-term facilities from the count, the number of short-term nonfederal hospitals increased by 3.6 percent over the decade, and the number of beds in these facilities rose 24.1 percent. Thus, for general health care of the public at large, there was a modest increase in facilities over the decade ending in 1973.

During the five-year period studied the number of short-term nonfederal hospitals rose by 1.2 percent, and the number of beds increased by 12.0 percent. Hospitals with less than a fifty-bed capacity represented 32 percent of all hospitals in 1968 and 27 percent in 1973; the number of such hospitals declined by 14.1 percent over the five-year period, and the number of beds in them declined by 14.6 percent. Larger hospitals—400 or more beds— represented 6.4 percent of all hospitals in 1968 and 8.2 percent in 1973. The number of such rose by 30 percent over the five-year period, and the number of beds in them increased by 23.3 percent. Larger hospitals were relatively more common in 1973 than in 1968.

While overall capacity of hospitals rose, the average length of stay dropped from 8.4 days in 1968 to 7.8 days in 1973, a decline of 7.1 percent; and the occupancy rate dropped from 78.2 percent to 75.4 percent over the five-year period, a decline of 3.6 percent. If one measures utilization by adjusting the occupancy rate for the change in the number of beds over the five years, the utilization of hospitals would show an increase rather than a decline. Such a computation shows an increase of 8.1 percent in hospital utilization.

From 1968 to 1973 the most significant change in the utilization of health care facilities across the nation occurred in the number of outpatient visits. There was a substantial increase in the use of hospital outpatient departments and other ambulatory health care facilities for primary health care. Total outpatient visits to hospitals increased by 56 percent from 1968 to 1973, a growth significantly larger than in any measure of inpatient service.

After the implementation of Medicare, the nursing and rest home industry experienced rapid growth. National data for the five-year period studied are not available, but the number of such homes rose by 32 percent from 1963 to 1971, and the number of beds increased by 111 percent over the same period.

Our findings in the Boston-Cambridge area did not differ significantly from most measures of utilization of national health care facilities—except that the number of short-term nonfederal hospitals remained about the same and the number of beds declined slightly (0.04 percent), compared with a rise of 12.0 percent in the number of beds nationwide. The average length of stay in hospitals remained slightly higher than the national average, but over the five-year period the length of stay dropped 2.6 percent, compared with a drop of 7.1 percent for the nation as a whole. The occupancy rate was higher in Boston-Cambridge hospitals and showed a slight increase, 2.2 percent, compared with a national decline of 3.6 percent.

Just as in the nation as a whole, there were substantial increases in the number of outpatient visits in health care facilities in Boston-Cambridge. During the five-year period studied outpatient visits in Boston-Cambridge increased by 31.4 percent, considerably less than the national figure of 56.0 percent.

In our survey area there was a 15 percent increase in the number of nursing and rest homes over the five-year period, and the number of beds in these facilities grew by 27.5 percent. The occupancy rates of these facilities remained high—94.1 percent in 1968 and 96.1 percent in 1973, an increase of 2.1 percent.

In general one may conclude that the change in utilization of health care facilities in the Boston-Cambridge area over the 1968-73 period did not differ significantly from the changes in the nation as a whole. On margin, the changes in Boston-Cambridge were probably not as large as the average changes elsewhere in the country. In view of the relatively close relationship between the utilization of facilities and employment, one could readily conclude that, if the modest increase in the utilization of facilities in Boston-Cambridge resulted in a rise in employment, then the larger increase in the nationwide utilization of facilities is likely to result in an even larger rise in health care employment throughout the nation.

## Utilization of Health Manpower

The total number of persons employed in the United States rose from 75.9 million in 1968 to 84.4 million in 1973, an increase of 11.2 percent. Employment in the health care industry in the United States grew considerably faster. In the twenty-one selected health occupations included in this study, estimated employment rose from 2.5 million in 1968 to over 3.0 million in 1973, an increase of 22.0 percent, double the increase in national employment.

Since the increase in utilization of health care facilities from 1968 to 1973 was somewhat greater for the total United States than for Boston-Cambridge, one would assume that health care employment for the nation would have risen faster. However, this was not the case. During the five-year period the level of employment in health facilities in Boston-Cambridge increased by 25.2 percent, slightly more than in the nation as a whole.

The Boston-Cambridge area has a relatively high concentration of health facilities, and the major ones are teaching hospitals affiliated with universities. Such university-affiliated facilities are more likely to institute new technology and to employ a higher ratio of health care employees per patient than other health facilities. These factors may have offset the smaller increases in utilization of health facilities in the Boston-Cambridge area.

Of the three major types of health employers in the survey area (hospitals, nursing and rest homes, and ambulatory facilities), hospitals were the largest, employing in 1973 about four out of every five health care employees. Hospital employment rose by 25.4 percent over the five-year period. Employment in nursing and rest homes showed a slight decline of 1.7 percent, while employment in ambulatory facilities showed a substantial increase of 97.8 percent.

All twenty-one selected health occupations in Boston-Cambridge showed employment increases over the five-year period. The largest percentage increases were shown in the occupations of nurse practitioner, physician's assistant, radiologic technician, social worker (B.A.), and inhalation therapist. Increases for the major occupations, excluding physicians, varied considerably, and some were substantial: registered nurse, 26.7 percent; licensed practical nurse, 2.8 percent; nurse's aide, 12.6 percent; medical technologist, 50.1 percent; and medical technician, 44.6 percent.

There is no general agreement within the industry as to which of the numerous occupations are entry-level jobs. In our judgment there are about twenty health occupations that can be used as entry-level positions, which comprise approximately 40 percent of total employment in the industry.

The most important entry-level position (in terms of number of employees) is that of nurse's aide. Employment of this occupation in hospitals increased by almost 14 percent, while licensed practical nurses and registered nurses showed gains of 17 and nearly 25 percent, respectively. In nursing and rest homes, nurse's aide was the only occupation that showed an increase over the five-year period.

## Employment Prospects for Health Workers

The principal purpose of this study was to determine whether employment and job opportunities in the health care industry had decreased over the five-year period from 1968 to 1973 as a result of the decline in hospital occupancy rates. Traditionally, hospital occupancy rates have been used as the principal measure of hospital utilization. Further investigation called into question whether the occupancy rate alone is an effective measure of how inpatient facilities have been used over time. Our research indicates that when other more reliable measures are included—such as the number of admissions and the average length of stay—overall hospital utilization actually increased during this period. Moreover, we conclude that the decline in the occupancy rate during the five-year period was due to the disproportionate increase in the number of beds, which exceeded actual increased demand for health services.

The focus has been on hospitals because they are the traditional health care provider and continue to employ eight out of every ten health workers in the twenty-one categories studied. Although the number of other health care providers, such as nursing and rest homes and ambulatory facilities, has grown, these alternative providers are far less labor-intensive than inpatient facilities, and they are relatively new on the health care scene. In summary, more health care has been demanded from a wide variety of providers, but hospitals have maintained their dominance. Their proportion of health care workers has remained stable.

A number of factors give some assurance that the trend of employment growth in the industry will continue: the labor-intensive nature of the industry; the rapid development in technology, which requires specially trained workers; and the continued emphasis on the new generation of health providers (ambulatory facilities, such as neighborhood health centers and clinics). The increasing demand for health care (in terms of both quantity and quality) will contribute to the growth rate in employment of health workers. These elements, which led to growth in the past are likely to lead to further expansion in all sectors of the industry. As a result, job opportunities in the health industry are likely to expand.

Two additional factors may have a very significant impact on the demand for health services and manpower. The first of these is the imminent adoption of national health insurance (NHI) in one form or another.[1]

Since the increased coverage will place considerable stress on inpatient facilities, the current surplus of beds will quickly disappear and more beds will be demanded. Outpatient care, which has not been included in most existing third-party coverage, will be emphasized whether covered or not in any NHI plan. It has been recognized that ambulatory facilities are the most appropriate source for the vast majority of primary health care, especially in inner-city neighborhoods. Moreover, ambulatory care could well absorb any possible excess demand for health care placed on inpatient facilities. Ambulatory facilities are most cost-effective, and less lead time is required to make such facilities operational.

The manpower implication of these possible results is an increase in demand for all categories of health workers by inpatient care facilities and an increase in demand for a somewhat more comprehensively trained health worker mix (adding pediatric nurse practitioners, for example) in ambulatory facilities.

The second factor is that the affluence of American society has meant a growing interest in more education, which in turn has increased the demand for health services. American consumers continue to seek more health services, but they are also more critical of the quality of services offered. This trend has already led to a more cautious practice of medicine by the industry (defensive medicine), which involves an increase in consultations, laboratory tests, and other auxiliary services. It also will undoubtedly mean a continued growth in the demand for health personnel.

The prospects are good for substantial increases in the demand for health manpower in the future, but there are no reliable estimates of how this growth will affect the various occupations and professions in the industry. If the growth in the demand for health manpower were to occur across the entire occupational structure, planning for it would be relatively easy. However, there are indications that structural changes are already taking place. As the nation's health goals and priorities change, so also will the demand for services change. And the impact on the demand for personnel could vary significantly among various groups of health occupations.

A substantial part of the growth in allied health occupations has been in functions that were at one time performed by physicians. When the demand for physicians' services expanded faster than the supply of practicing physicians, the rate of permissible encroachment by allied health personnel on the functions of physicians increased. In recent years there has been an acceleration of this process, as the increase in the number of practicing physicians failed even to keep pace with the population growth. Some specific physician functions are now assigned to new allied health occupations (such as PNPs and physician's assistants) and are generally performed under the indirect supervision of the physicians. Need for other such health occupations could well develop in the future. In addition, many existing occupations continue to acquire functions that have traditionally been performed by physicians.

If the projected growth rate in the demand for health services materializes, there will be increased demand for nearly all health occupations. The shortage of practicing physicians will be especially acute. We conclude that the shortage will have two major effects on the structure of health manpower. First, the lead time required to train physicians and highly skilled workers, plus the institutional barriers limiting supply, will force a relatively greater utilization of less highly trained health personnel. For example, as registered nurses assume more sophisticated medical tasks, there will be increased opportunities for upward mobility from entry-level nursing positions.

As a result, the occupations described as entry-level or near-entry-level will have the greatest potential for growth. Since a large proportion of the employment in the industry could be considered near-entry-level, such expansion could very well provide many job opportunities, particularly for the disadvantaged. In the past, institutional barriers have excluded the disadvantaged or restricted them to dead-end jobs. In spite of recent progress in this area, it is apparent that the disadvantaged person—who may be black, Spanish-speaking, or a high school drop-out—has not participated in full measure in this rapidly growing field.

For the industry as a whole, the future looks bright. This general conclusion is predicated on the following factors:

1. the current growth rates of inpatient facilities in hospitals; outpatient facilities, either hospital-based or not; and nursing and rest homes;

2. the continued development and adoption of sophisticated health care technology;

3. the continued trend toward specialization among health workers as a result of new technology;

4. the expansion of the practice of defensive medicine in face of increasing vigilance of the American consumer of health care;

5. the gradual but continuous absorption of physician functions by allied health personnel;

6. the increased demand for health services in general, brought about by the increasing affluence of the American public as well as by the growth in the total population;

7. the expected passage of a national health insurance program.

The general conclusion we must draw is that there still is a substantial need for education and training programs for the whole range of allied health occupations, especially for occupations at the lower and middle levels of the range.

# Notes

## CHAPTER 1

1. David D. Rutstein, *The Coming Revolution in Medicine* (Cambridge: MIT Press, 1967), pp. 9-48.

2. U.S. Department of Health, Education and Welfare, Social Security Administration, *Calendar 1972 Highlights,* by Barbara S. Cooper, Nancy L. Worthington, and Paula A. Piro, Pub. No. 11701 (Washington: Government Printing Office, 1974), p. 2.

3. United Nations, *Statistical Yearbook, 1974* (New York: United Nations, 1975), pp. 80-85.

4. *Ibid.*

5. U.S. Department of Commerce, Bureau of the Census, *Statistical Abstract of the United States 1974* (Washington: Government Printing Office, 1974), pp. 58, 60.

6. *Ibid.,* p. 58. This 71.2 years is an average of the 67.4 years for males and 75.2 years for females.

7. Marjorie Smith Mueller and Robert M. Gibson, "National Health Expenditures, Fiscal Year 1975," *Social Security Bulletin* 39:2, p. 6.

8. U.S. Department of Health, Education and Welfare, Social Security Administration, *Research and Statistics,* Note No. 18, "Projections of National Health Expenditures, 1975 and 1980," by Dorothy P. Rice and Mary F. McGee (Washington: Government Printing Office, October 1970).

9. *Ibid.*

10. Center for Health Policy Studies, *Chartbook of Federal Health Spending* (Washington: National Planning Association, 1974), p. 20.

11. *Ibid.,* p. 21-22.

12. *Ibid.,* p. 23.

13. United Nations, *Statistical Yearbook, 1974,* pp. 644-649.

14. Center for Health Policy Studies, *Chartbook of Federal Health Spending*, p. 2.

15. *Ibid.*, p. 3; and U.S. Department of Health, Education and Welfare, Social Security Administration, *Compendium of National Health Expenditure Data*, by Barbara S. Cooper, Nancy Worthington, and Mary McGee (Washington: Government Printing Office, 1972), pp. 51-54.

16. Committee for Economic Development, *Building a National Health Care System* (New York: Committee for Economic Development, April 1973), p. 14.

17. U.S. Department of Health, Education and Welfare, National Center for Health Statistics, *Health Resources Statistics*, 1974 (Washington: Government Printing Office, 1975).

18. Unpublished estimates from U.S. Department of Health, Education and Welfare, National Center for Health Statistics, January 1976.

19. Dean S. Ammer, *Institutional Employment and Shortage of Paramedical Personnel: A Detailed Study of Staffing in Hospitals, Nursing Homes, and Various Institutions in the Greater Boston Area* (Boston: Northeastern University, 1967), p. V.

20. Eli Ginzberg with Miriam Ostow, *Men, Money, and Medicine* (New York: Columbia University Press, 1969), pp. 133-134.

21. Committee for Economic Development, *Building a National Health Care System*, p. 33.

22. Ginzberg with Ostow, *Men, Money, and Medicine*, p. 64.

23. U.S. Department of Labor, Bureau of Labor Statistics, *Annual Earnings and Employment Patterns of Private Non-agricultural Employees, 1965*, Bulletin 1675 (Washington: Government Printing Office, 1970), Table 1, pp. 9-10; and *Industry Wage Survey, Hospitals, March 1969* Bulletin 1688 (Washington: Government Printing Office, 1971), pp. 14-15.

24. Vicente Navarro, "Health and Corporate Society," *Social Policy*, January/February 1975, p. 92.

25. See U.S. Bureau of the Census, *Statistical Abstracts 1974*, pp. 353-356.

# CHAPTER 3

1. Milton I. Roemer and Jay W. Friedman, *Doctors in Hospitals* (Baltimore: Johns Hopkins Press, 1971), p. 34.

2. Abraham Flexner, *Medical Education in the United States and Canada*, Bulletin No. 4, Carnegie Foundation for the Advancement of Teaching, 1910.

3. U.S. Department of Commerce, Bureau of the Census, *Statistical Abstract 1975* (Washington: Government Printing Office, 1975), p. 70.

4. *Ibid.*

5. U.S. Department of Health, Education and Welfare, Social Security Administration, *Calendar 1972 Highlights*, by Barbara S. Cooper, Nancy L. Worthington, and Paula A. Piro, Pub. No. 11701 (Washington: Government Printing Office, 1974), p. 3.

6. American Hospital Association, *Hospital Statistics*, 1974 (Chicago: American Hospital Association, 1974), p. 7.

7. Harold M. Goldstein, "Health and Medical Care," in *The Economist Looks at Society,* edited by Gustav Schacter and Edwin L. Dale, Jr. (Lexington, Massachusetts: Zerox, 1973), p. 165.

8. William J. Bicknell and Diana C. Walsh, "Certification-of-Need: The Massachusetts Experience," *New England Journal of Medicine* Vol. 292, May 15, 1975, pp. 1054-1061.

9. *Ibid.*

# CHAPTER 4

1. In Massachusetts the Department of Public Health classifies nursing and rest homes in four separate categories. See Appendix D.

2. U.S. Department of Health, Education and Welfare, National Center for Health Statistics, *Vital and Health Statistics,* Series 12, No. 19, "Characteristics of Residents in Nursing and Personal Care Homes—June-August 1969." (Washington: Government Printing Office, 1972).

3. U.S. Department of Health, Education and Welfare, National Center for Health Statistics, *Monthly Vital Statistics Report,* "1973-74 Nursing Home Survey: Provisional Data," Pub. No. HRA 75-1120 (Washington: Government Printing Office, 1974), p. 3.

4. U.S. Department of Health, Education and Welfare, National Center for Health Statistics, *Health Resources Statistics,* 1974 (Washington: Government Printing Office, 1975), p. 383.

5. *Ibid.,* p. 382.

6. Ibid., p. 395.

7. Craig Stuart and H. Lee Barrett, Jr., "Medicaid and Boston's Neighborhood Health Centers: Integrating Two Concepts of Health Care," unpublished paper, p. 63.

8. *Ibid.,* p. 80.

9. See letter to the *Boston Globe* from Thomas F. Sullivan, Assistant Regional Director of Health, DHEW Region I, March 28, 1973.

# CHAPTER 5

1. We limited employment to health care occupations, omitting such groups as dieticians, kitchen help, custodial and protection employees, as well as building maintenance occupations, even though employment in these occupations may represent a significant percentage of the industry's total employment.

2. U.S. Department of Health, Education and Welfare, National Center for Health Statistics, *Health Resource Statistics,* 1974 (Washington: Government Printing Office, 1975), pp. 9-14.

# CHAPTER 7

1. For a detailed discussion of the possible effects of alternative insurance plans on the demand for service and manpower, see Joseph P. Newhouse, Charles E. Phelps, and William B. Schwartz, "Policy Options and the Impact of National Health Insurance," *New England Journal of Medicine* June 13, 1974, No. 290, pp. 1345-1359.

# Appendix A

# CMMS Letter

(See overleaf, page 104.)

COLLEGE OF LIBERAL ARTS
DEPARTMENT OF ECONOMICS

December 15, 1974

Dear Sir:

This letter is to introduce the Center for Medical Manpower Studies, located at Northeastern University. Since 1967 we have worked on various research grants funded by the U.S. Department of Labor, Manpower Administration and the National Institutes of Health in the field of allied health manpower. Currently we are involved in a project entitled, "Health Manpower Employment in Boston and Cambridge."

Over the past ten years, there has been an increase in demand for health services accompanied by an increase in the types of providers. Many of the facilities that now are treating the "vertical patient" were not in existence in 1968 and 1971. These newly licensed facilities are competing with one another for certain allied health personnel to provide increased services. Your facility has probably felt this competition and our study is interested in learning how you have coped with it. How do you attract personnel to your facility and how do you retain them? These are some of the questions and problems with which our project is dealing.

Part of our research entails contacting all health providers in the Boston and Cambridge area. Basically we are looking for numbers of health personnel employed in ambulatory facilities as well as some indication of utilization, i.e., number of visits, cases, encounters for the years 1968, 1971 and 1973. We are also cooperating with the State Office of Manpower Affairs and the Massachusetts Department of Public Health which has undertaken a similar project.

If your facility was in operation in 1968, 1971 or 1973 we would very much appreciate your cooperation. Enclosed is a copy of our questionnaire. A member of the Center's staff will contact you by telephone in the near future to make arrangements to collect this information at your convenience.

Thank you in advance for your cooperation.

Sincerely,

Harold M. Goldstein
Professor and Director

CENTER FOR MEDICAL MANPOWER STUDIES

104

# Appendix B

## CMMS Questionnaire

Name of Facility: _____

Questionnaire Completed by: Name: _____

Phone No. _____

The Center for Medical Manpower Studies, Northeastern University, is gathering the information indicated below (the growth of various allied health occupations employed in Boston and Cambridge between 1968 and 1973) under the auspices of the Manpower Administration, U.S. Department of Labor. We would appreciate it if you would complete the following page for your facility using end of either fiscal or calendar year data according to the following guidelines:

Full-Time Employees—Employee on payroll who works 35 or more hours per week.
Part-Time Employee—Employee on payroll who works less than 35 hours per week.

| Number of Health Workers in the Following Categories Employed | 1968 | | 1971 | | 1973 | |
|---|---|---|---|---|---|---|
| | FT | PT | FT | PT | FT | PT |
| Intern, Resident | | | | | | |
| All Other Physicians | | | | | | |
| Nurse Practitioner or Pediatric Nurse Practitioner | | | | | | |
| Physician's Assistant | | | | | | |
| Registered Nurse | | | | | | |
| Licensed Practical Nurse | | | | | | |
| Nurse's Aide/Orderly | | | | | | |
| Nurse Anesthetist | | | | | | |
| Pharmacist | | | | | | |
| Radiologic Technician | | | | | | |
| Medical Technologist (MT) | | | | | | |
| Medical Technician (CLA) | | | | | | |
| OR Technician | | | | | | |
| Physical Therapist | | | | | | |
| Physical Therapist's Assistant | | | | | | |
| Social Worker (B.A.) | | | | | | |
| Social Worker (M.S.W.) | | | | | | |
| Inhalation Therapist | | | | | | |
| Speech Therapist | | | | | | |
| EKG Technician | | | | | | |
| EEG Technician | | | | | | |

If you have any questions about the questionnaire please write or call: Pat McCarville or Kathy Calore, Center for Medical Manpower Studies, Dept. of Economics, Northeastern University, Boston, Mass. 02115. Tel: 437-3640 or 437-2884.

## Appendix C

## Occupations and Descriptions[1]

*Intern, Resident* Graduates of an approved medical school who are enrolled in formal hospital training programs. The internship is necessary in thirty-four states and the District of Columbia in order to be licensed. To become certified specialists, physicians must pass specialty board examinations. To qualify for these exams they must spend between two and four years, depending on the specialty, in advanced hospital training as resident.

*All Other Physicians* Most medical schools require applicants to have completed at least three years of college education; some require four years. Most students who enter medical schools have a bachelor's degree. All states and the District of Columbia require a license to practice medicine. A physician must graduate from an approved school of medicine, pass a licensing exam, and in thirty-four states and the District of Columbia, complete a one-year hospital internship. Licensing examinations are given by state boards. The National Board of Medical Examiners also gives an examination, which is accepted by forty-eight states and the District of Columbia as a substitute for state examinations.

*Nurse Practitioner, Pediatric Nurse Practitioner* Registered nurses who, with extra training, prepare for highly independent roles in the clinical care and teaching of patients. They practice in primary roles that include nurse-midwifery, maternal care, pediatrics, family health, and the care of medical patients. The nurse practitioner programs consist of classroom instruction and clinical experience lasting about three months.

*Physician's Assistant*   The assistant to a primary care physician is a skilled person qualified by academic and clinical training to provide patient services under the supervision and responsibility of a physician. The physician's assistant performs diagnostic and therapeutic tasks in order to allow a physician to extend his or her services through the more effective use of knowledge, skills, and abilities.

*Registered Nurse*   Professional nurses are trained in one of three programs. Diploma programs are conducted by hospitals and independent schools and usually require three years of training. Bachelor degree programs usually require four years of study in a college or university, although a few require five years. Associate degree programs in junior and community colleges require approximately two years of nursing education. A license is required in all states to practice as a professional nurse.

*Licensed Practical Nurse*   Working under the direction of physicians and nurses, they provide nursing care that requires technical knowledge but not the professional training of a registered nurse. All states and the District of Columbia regulate the preparation and licensing of practical nurses. To be licensed, students must complete a course of instruction in practical nursing that has been approved by the state board of nursing and pass a licensing examination. Educational requirements for enrollment in state-approved training programs range from completion of eighth grade to high school graduation. Practical nurse programs are generally one year long and include both classroom study and clinical practice.

*Nurse's Aide, Orderly*   The duties of nurse's aides depend on the policies of the institutions where they work. Some institutions require high school diplomas, but many hire nongraduates. Nurse's aides generally are trained after they are hired. Some institutions combine on-the-job training, under the close supervision of registered or licensed practical nurses, and classroom instruction. Training may last several days or a few months. Without further training, opportunities for promotion are limited. (Also called hospital attendant, nursing assistant, auxiliary nursing worker, home health aide.)

*Nurse Anesthetist*   Nurse anesthetists are licensed professional nurses who have completed an approved program for nurse anesthetists. They are accredited by the American Association of Nurse Anesthetists.

*Pharmacist*   Pharmacists dispense drugs and medicines prescribed by medical practitioners. A license to practice pharmacy is required in all states and the District of Columbia. To obtain a license, one must be a graduate of an accredited pharmacy college, pass a state board examination, and have a specified amount of practical experience or internship under the supervision of a registered pharmacist. In general, five or six years of study beyond high school are required.

*Radiologic (X-Ray) Technician*   They operate X-ray equipment, usually under the supervision of a radiologist. Some do radiation therapy work and others work in the field of nuclear medicine. The requirement for entry into this field is the completion of a formal training program in X-ray technology, generally offered in hospitals, medical schools, and colleges. Some courses in X-ray technology are offered by vocational or technical schools. Programs usually take twenty-four months to complete. A few offer three- or four-year programs, and about thirty schools award a bachelor's degree in X-ray technology. (Also called radiologic technologist, X-ray technician, X-ray technologist.)

*Medical Technologist*   Medical technologists perform various chemical, microscopic, bacteriologic, and related tests. They require four years of college training, including completion of a specialized training program in medical technology. A medical technologist may be certified as Medical Technologist, MT (ASCP) by the American Society of Clinical Pathologists; Medical Technologist, MT, by the American Medical Technologists; or Registered Medical Technologist, RMT, by the International Society of Clinical Laboratory Technologists. (Also called blood bank technologist, chemistry technologist, hematology technologist.)

*Medical Technician*  Medical technicians require two years of postsecondary training to perform a wide range of tests and laboratory procedures that require a high level of skill but not the technical knowledge of the highly trained technologists. Medical laboratory technicians can be trained in a variety of settings. Medical technicians must be licensed in nine states, New York City, and Puerto Rico.

*OR Technician*  Operating room technicians assist surgeons and anesthesiologists before, during, and after surgery. They are supervised by registered nurses. Most operating room technicians are trained on the job. A high school education or equivalent is generally required for employment. On-the-job training programs in many hospitals include classroom instruction. The length of these programs varies from six weeks to one year, depending on the trainee's qualifications and the training given. (Also called surgical technician.)

*Physical Therapist*  Physical therapists assist individuals with muscle, nerve, joint, and bone diseases or injuries to overcome their resulting disabilities. All states and the District of Columbia require a license to practice physical therapy. Applicants for a license must have a degree or certificate from a school of physical therapy, and to qualify they must pass a state board examination. Most approved schools offer bachelor's degree programs, but some provide one- to two-year programs.

*Physical Therapist's Assistant*  Physical therapist's assistants work under the supervision of professional physical therapists to restore physical functions and prevent disability from injury or illness. Fourteen states (in 1972) licensed physical therapist's assistants who had completed an approved two-year associate degree program.

*Social Worker (B.A.)*  A bachelor's degree is the minimum educational requirement for entry-level jobs in social work. The functions of a social worker (B.A.) are similar to those of a social worker (M.S.W.).

*Social Worker (M.S.W.)*  A social worker (M.S.W.) must have earned a master's degree in social work by completing two years of specialized study and supervised field instruction. Social workers in medical and psychiatric settings aid patients, families, and communities with social problems that accompany illness, recovery, and rehabilitation. As members of a medical team, they help patients respond to treatment and guide them in their readjustment to their homes, jobs, and communities.

*Inhalation Therapist, Inhalation Technician, Respiratory Therapist* Persons with these job titles perform essentially the same duties, although the therapist is expected to have a higher level of expertise and may be expected to assume some teaching and supervisory duties. Duties range from giving temporary relief to patients with chronic asthma to giving emergency care in cases of heart failure, stroke, and shock. Formal courses in inhalation therapy vary in length between eighteen months and four years and include both theory and clinical work. Respiratory therapists with associate's degrees from a program approved by the American Medical Association and one year of experience are eligible to be registered by the American Registry of Inhalation Therapists. In addition, there are a few therapists who are trained on the job. However, formal training as a requisite to entering the field is being stressed as respiratory apparatus becomes more complex.

*Speech Pathologist* Speech pathologists diagnose and administer therapy for speech and language problems. They must have at least a bachelor's degree in speech pathology. In eighteen states speech pathologists are required to have a license to practice, and those who are licensed must have a master's degree in speech pathology, complete 300 hours of clinical practicum with a certified speech therapist, and pass a written examination. The American Speech and Hearing Association certifies graduates who have completed a master's degree in speech pathology, worked with a certified speech pathologist for 300 hours of clinical practicum, and completed a year's intensive work under the supervision of a certified speech pathologist.

*Electrocardiograph (EKG) Technician* Electrocardiograph technicians take and process electrocardiograms at the request of a physician. EKG technicians generally are trained on the job. Training, which may last as long as three months, is usually conducted by a senior EKG technician or a cardiologist. The minimum requirement for the job usually is a high school diploma. The military services also train EKG technicians.

*Electroencephalographic (EEG) Technician*   Electroencephalographic technicians perform the EEG procedure and maintain the equipment. Most EEG technicians are trained on the job by experienced EEG personnel. There are some formal training programs in colleges and medical schools, which range from six months to two years in length. EEG technicians who have one year of training and one year of experience and who successfully complete a written and oral examination administered by the American Board of Registration of Electroencephalograph Technologists may become registered.

---

[1]Two sources for these descriptions are U.S. Department of Labor, Bureau of Labor Statistics, *Occupational Outlook Handbook,* 1974-75 edition, Bulletin 1785; and American Hospital Association, Council on Medical Education, *Allied Medical Education Directory,* 1973.

# Appendix D

## Definition of Levels of Care for Nursing and Rest Homes in Massachusetts

**Facilities that provide Level I care shall provide:**

    a. A full-time director of nurses.
    b. A full-time supervisor of nurses during the day shift.
    c. A charge nurse 24 hours per day, seven days a week.
    d. Sufficient ancillary nursing personnel to meet patient needs.
    e. 2.6 hours of nursing care per patient per day; 0.6 hours shall be provided by licensed nursing personnel and 2.0 hours by ancillary nursing personnel.

**Facilities that provide Level II care shall provide:**

    a. A full-time director of nurses.
    b. A charge nurse 24 hours per day.
    c. Sufficient ancillary nursing personnel to meet patient needs.
    d. 2.0 hours of nursing care per patient per day; 0.6 hours shall be provided by licensed nursing personnel and 1.4 hours by ancillary nursing personnel.

113

**Facilities that provide Level III care shall provide:**

a. A full-time supervisor of nurses during the day shift, five days a week.

b. A charge nurse during the day and evening shifts, seven days a week.

c. A nurse's aide who is a responsible person, on duty during the night shift.

d. Sufficient ancillary nursing personnel to meet patient needs.

e. 1.4 hours of nursing care per patient day; 0.4 hours shall be provided by licensed nursing personnel and 1.0 hours by ancillary personnel.


**Facilities that provide Level IV care shall provide:**

a. In facilities with less than 20 beds, at least one "responsible" person" on *active* duty during the waking hours in the ratio of one per ten residents.

b. In facilities with more than 20 beds, at least one "responsible person" on *active* duty at all time during the 24 hours of the day.

c. If none of the responsible persons on duty are licensed nurses, then the facility shall provide a licensed consultant nurse, four hours per month per unit.

Source: *Rules and Regulations for the Licensing of Long-Term Care Facilities* (Boston: Massachusetts Department of Public Health, Division of Medical Care, Bureau of Health Facilities, 1971), pp. 18-20.

# Selected Bibliography

Alevizos, Gus; Walsh, Robert J.; and Aherne, Phil. *Socioeconomic Issues of Health.* Center for Health Services Research and Development. Chicago: American Medical Association, 1973.

American Hospital Association. *Hospitals,* Guide Issues. Chicago: American Hospital Association, annual, 1950-74.

———. *Survey of Hospital Charges as of January 1, 1974.* Chicago: American Hospital Association, 1974.

———. *Hospital Statistics.* Chicago: American Hospital Association, annual, 1972, 1973, 1974.

American Medical Association. *Allied Medical Education Directory, 1973.* Chicago: American Medical Association, 1973.

———. *Medical Education in the United States 1972-1973.* Reprinted from *Journal of the American Medical Association,* 226, 8 (November 19, 1973). Chicago: American Medical Association, 1973.

American Medical Association, Council on Medical Education. *Allied Medical Education Directory 1973.* Chicago: American Medical Association, 1973.

Ammer, Dean S. *Institutional Employment and Shortages of Paramedical Personnel: A Detailed Study of Staffing in Hospitals, Nursing Homes, and Various Institutions in the Greater Boston Area.* Grant from U.S. Public Health Service. Boston: Northeastern University, 1967.

Anderson, Odin W. *Health Care: Can There be Equity? The United States, Sweden, and England.* New York: John Wiley & Sons, 1972.

Baehr, George. "Some Popular Delusions About Health and Medical Care." *American Journal of Public Health* (March 1971), 582-586.

115

Baird, Charles W. "On Profits and Hospitals." *Journal of Economic Issues* Vol. V, No. 1 (March 1971), 57-67.

Berg, Robert L., M.D., ed. *Health Status Indexes.* Chicago: Hospital Research and Educational Trust, 1973.

Berki, Sylvester E. *Hospital Economics.* Lexington, Massachusetts: D.C. Heath and Co., Lexington Books, 1972.

Bicknell, William J., M.D., and Walsh, Diana C. "Certification-of-Need: The Massachusetts Experience," *New England Journal of Medicine* Vol. CCVIIIC (May 15, 1975), 1054-1061.

Burns, Eveline M. *Health Services for Tomorrow.* New York: Dunellen Publishing Co., 1973.

Committee for Economic Development. *Building a National Health Care System.* New York: Committee for Economic Development, April 1973.

Connecticut Institute for Health Manpower Resources, Inc. *Study of Educational Programs and Employment Opportunities in Health in Connecticut and the Northeast.* Hartford: Connecticut Institute for Health Manpower Resources, 1974.

Densen, Paul M. "Medical Schools and the Delivery of Medical Care to the Community." *New England Journal of Medicine* (May 20, 1971), 1156-1157.

DMI Health Manpower Information Exchange. *Documents Related to Health Manpower Planning: A Bibliography.* Preliminary Report. Washington: Government Printing Office, 1974.

Doyle, Patrick J., M.D. *Save Your Health and Your Money.* Washington: Acropolis Books, 1971.

Eilers, Robert D. "National Health Insurance: What Kind and How Much." *New England Journal of Medicine* (April 22, 1971), 881-887; (April 29, 1971), 945-955.

Fein, Rashi. "Can the 'Doctor Shortage' Be Solved?" *Hospital Practice* (April 1971), 73-101.

_____. *The Doctor Shortage.* Washington, D.C.: Brookings Institution, 1967.

Fein, Rashi, and Weber, Gerald I. *Financing Medical Education.* A general report prepared for The Carnegie Commission on Higher Education and the Commonwealth Fund. New York: McGraw-Hill, 1971.

Flexner, Abraham. *Medical Education in the United States and Canada.* Commissioned by the Carnegie Foundation for the Advancement of Teaching, 1910. Reprint. Washington: Science and Health Publications, 1960.

Freeman, Howard E.; Levine, Sol; and Reeder, Leo G. *Handbook of Medical Sociology.* 2d ed. Englewood, New Jersey: Prentice-Hall, 1972.

Fuchs, Victor R. *Who Shall Live?* New York: Basic Books, 1974.

Ginzberg, Eli; and the Conservation of Human Resources Staff, Columbia University. *Urban Health Services: The Case of New York.* New York: Columbia University Press, 1971.

Ginzberg, Eli, with Ostow, Miriam. *Men, Money, and Medicine.* New York: Columbia University Press, 1969.

Goldstein, Harold M. "Health and Medical Care," in *The Economist Looks at Society,* edited by Gustav Schachter and Edwin L. Dale, Jr. Lexington, Massachusetts : Xerox, 1973.

Gorman, Mike. "The Impact of National Health Insurance on Delivery of Health Care." *American Journal of Public Health* (May 1971), 962-972.

Greenfield, Harry I. *Hospital Efficiency and Public Policy.* Center for Policy Research. New York: Praeger, 1973.

Grossman, Michael. *The Demand for Health: A Theoretical and Empirical Investigation.* National Bureau of Economic Research, Occasional Paper 119. New York: Columbia University Press, 1972.

Keeler, Emmett B.; Newhouse, Joseph P.; and Phelps, Charles E. *Deductibles and the Demand for Medical Services: The Theory of the Consumer Facing a Variable Price Schedule Under Uncertainty.* Santa Monica: Rand Corporation, 1974.

Krizay, John, and Wilson, Andrew. *The Patient As Consumer.* A Twentieth Century Fund Report. Lexington, Massachusetts: D.C. Heath and Co., Lexington Books, 1974.

Lerner, Monroe, and Anderson, Odin W. *Health Progress in the United States: 1900-1960.* A Report of the Health Information Foundation. Chicago: University of Chicago Press, 1963.

Levey, Samuel, and Loomba, N. Paul. *Health Care Administration.* Philadelphia: J.B. Lippincott Co., 1973.

Luongo, Edward P., M.D. *American Medicine in Crisis.* New York: Philosophical Library, 1971.

Massachusetts, Commonwealth of. Department of Public Health. *Health Data Annual,* 1974, Vol. I, No. 1. Boston: Massachusetts Department of Public Health, 1974.

_____. Department of Public Health. Division of Medical Care. Bureau of Health Facilities. *Rules and Regulations for the Licensing of Long-Term Care Facilities.* Boston: Massachusetts Department of Public Health, 1971.

_____. Executive Office for Administration and Finance. *Massachusetts Inventory of Published Statistical Series.* Boston, 1970.

McCleery, Robert S., M.D. *One Life—One Physician.* Washington: Public Affairs Press, 1971.

McCormick, James B., and Kopp, Joseph B. "Manpower Consideration/Use of Technicians Frees Physicians." *Hospitals* (March 1971), 71-75.

McKinlay, John B., ed. *Economic Aspects of Health Care*. Milbank Memorial Fund. New York: Prodist, 1973.

Mendelson, Mary Adelaide. *Tender Loving Greed*. New York: Alfred A. Knopf, 1974.

Morreale, Joseph C., ed. *The U.S. Medical Care Industry: The Economist's Point of View*. Michigan Business Papers Number 60. Ann Arbor: University of Michigan, 1974.

Mueller, Marjorie Smith, and Gibson, Robert M. "National Health Expenditures, Fiscal Year 1975." *Social Security Bulletin* XXXIX, No. 2, 18.

National Academy of Sciences. *Costs of Education in the Health Professions, Parts I, II, and III*. Washington: Government Printing Office, 1974.

National Planning Association. Center for Health Policy Studies. *Chartbooks of Federal Health Spending*. Washington: Government Printing office, 1974.

Navarro, Vincente. "Health and Corporate Society." *Social Policy* (January/February 1975), 41.

Newhouse, Joseph P. *Forecasting Demand for Medical Care for the Purpose of Planning Health Services*. Santa Monica: Rand Corporation, 1974.

Newhouse, Joseph P., and Phelps, Charles E. *On Having Your Cake and Eating It Too: Econometric Problems in Estimating the Demand for Health Services*. Santa Monica: Rand Corporation, 1974.

Newhouse, Joseph P.; Phelps, Charles E.; and Schwartz, William B. "Policy Options and the Impact of National Health Insurance." *New England Journal of Medicine* (June 13, 1974), 1345-1359.

Organization for Economic and Community Development. *New Directions in Education for Changing Health Systems*. Paris: OECD, 1975.

Penchansky, Roy, ed. *Health Services Administration*. Cambridge: Harvard University Press, 1968.

Perlman, Mark, ed. *The Economics of Health and Medical Care*. New York: John Wiley & Sons, 1974.

Pharmaceutical Manufacturers Association. *Fact Book*. Washington: Pharmaceutical Manufacturers Association, 1972.

Phelps, Charles E. *Demand for Health Insurance: A Theoretical and Empirical Investigation*. Santa Monica: Rand Corporation, 1973.

Phelps, Charles E., and Newhouse, Joseph P. *Coinsurance and the Demand for Medical Services*. Santa Monica: Rand Corporation, 1974.

Pratt, Lois. "The Relationship of Socio-Economic Status to Health." *American Journal of Public Health* (February 1971), 281-292.

Rice, Dorothy P., and McGee, Mary F. "Projections of National Health Expenditures, 1975 and 1980." *Research and Statistics*, Note No. 18 (October 30, 1970). Washington: Government Printing Office, 1970.

Roemer, Milton I., and Friedman, Jay W. *Doctors in Hospitals.* Baltimore: Johns Hopkins Press, 1971.

Rosenberg, William E. "Who's Out of Date?" *New England Journal of Medicine* (April 15, 1971), 850-851.

Rutstein, David D., M.D. *The Coming Revolution in Medicine.* Cambridge: MIT Press, 1974.

_____. *Blueprint for Medical Care.* Cambridge: MIT Press, 1974.

Schechter, Daniel S. *Agenda for Continuing Education.* Chicago: Hospital Research and Educational Trust, 1974.

Scott, W. Richard, and Volkart, Edmund H., eds. *Medical Care Readings in the Sociology of Medical Institutions.* New York: John Wiley & Sons, 1966.

Sidenstricker, Edgar. *The Challenge of Facts: Selected Public Health Papers.* Edited by Richard V. Kasius. Milbank Memorial Fund. New York: Prodist, 1974.

Sigerist, Henry E. *On the Sociology of Medicine.* Edited by Milton I. Roemer, M.D. New York: MD Publications, 1960.

Skolik, Alfred M., and Dales, Sophie R. "Social Welfare Expenditures, 1968-1969." *Social Security Bulletin* XXXII (December 1969), 12.

Somers, Herman M., and Somers, Anne R. *Medicare and the Hospitals.* Washington: Brookings Institution, 1967.

Sorkin, Alan L. *Health Economics.* Lexington, Massachusetts: D.C. and Co., Lexington Books, 1975.

Steward, Charles T., Jr. "Allocations of Resources to Health." *Journal of Human Resources* (Winter 1971), 103-123.

Stuart, Craig, and Barrett, H. Lee, Jr. "Medicaid and Boston's Neighborhood Health Centers: Integrating Two Concepts of Health Care." Unpublished paper submitted to Professor Lloyd L. Weinre for Seminar on Institutional Change in Urban America, Harvard University, April 1972.

*Study of Accreditation of Selected Health Educational Programs.* Commission Report. Washington: National Commission on Accrediting, 1972.

Tribble, William D. *Doctor Draft Justified.* San Antonio, Texas: National Biomedical Laboratories, 1968.

United Nations Statistical Office. *Statistical Yearbook.* New York: United Nations, annual, 1972, 1974.

U.S. Department of Commerce. *Business Statistics, 1973.* Washington: Government Printing Office, 1973.

_____. *Survey of Current Business,* LIV, 4. Washington: Government Printing Office, 1974.

_____. Bureau of the Census. *Census of Population: 1970,* Vol. I, PC(1)-D1, United States Summary, Detailed Characteristics. Washington: Government Printing Office, 1970.

_____. *Statistical Abstract of the United States,* 1974. Washington: Government Printing Office, 1973 and 1974.

U.S. Department of Health, Education and Welfare. National Center for Health Statistics. *Characteristics of Residents in Nursing and Personal Care Homes, United States—June-August 1969.* Vital and Health Statistics, Series 12, Number 19. Washington: Government Printing Office, 1973.

_____. *Charges for Care in Nursing Homes: United States—April-September 1968.* Vital and Health Statistics, Series 12, Number 14. Washington. Government Printing Office, 1972.

_____. *Employees in Nursing Homes: United States—April September 1968.* Vital and Health Statistics, Series 12, Number 15. Washington: Government Printing Office, 1972.

_____. *Health Manpower Source Book 21.* Washington: Government Printing Office, 1970.

_____. *Health Resources Statistics.* Washington: Government Printing office, annual, 1969, 1972, 1973, 1974.

_____. "1973-74 Nursing Home Survey: Provisional Data." Monthly Vital Statistics Report, HRA 75-1120. Washington: Government Printing Office, 1974.

_____. *Selected Characteristics of Nursing Homes for the Aged and Chronically Ill: United States—June-August 1969.* Vital and Health Statistics, Series 12, Number 23. Washington: Government Printing Office, 1974.

_____. *Utilization of Institutions for the Aged and Chronically Ill: United States—April-June 1963.* Vital and Health Statistics, Series 12, Number 4. Washington: Government Printing Office, 1966.

U.S. Department of Health, Education and Welfare. Social Security Administration. *Calendar 1972 Highlights.* By Barbara S. Cooper, Nancy L. Worthington, and Paula Piro. Washington: Government Printing Office, 1974.

_____. *Compendium of National Health Expenditure Data.* By Barbara S. Cooper, Nancy Worthington, and Mary McGee. Washington: Government Printing Office, 1972.

_____. *Health Insurance Statistics,* 1968-72. Washington: Government Printing Office, annual.

_____. *Research and Statistics.* Note No. 3, 1973. Washington: Government Printing Office, 1973.

_____. *Social Security Bulletin,* December 1972. Washington: Government Printing Office, 1972.

U.S. Department of Labor; and U.S. Department of Health, Education and Welfare. *Manpower Report of the President,* 1974. Washington: Government Printing Office, 1974.

U.S. Department of Labor. Bureau of Labor Statistics. *Annual Earnings*

*and Employment Patterns of Private Non-Agricultural Employees,*
1965. Bulletin 1675. Washington: Government Printing Office, 1971.

————. *Consumer Price Index for Selected Items and Groups,*
*Monthly and Annual Averages.* Washington: Government Printing
Office, annual, 1950-72.

————. *Employment and Earnings.* Washington: Government Printing Office, monthly, 1950-73.

————. "Employment in the Medical and Other Health Services."
Based on unpublished data from U.S. Department of Commerce, *Statistical Abstract of the United States* 1973, Table No. 107.

————. *Industry and Wage Survey, Hospitals,* March 1969. Bulletin
1688. Washington: Government Printing Office: 1971.

————. *Occupational Outlook Handbook,* 1974-75 edition. Washington: Government Printing Office, 1974.

————. *Occupational Outlook Quarterly,* Vol. XIV, No. 4. Washington: Government Printing Office, 1970.

————. *Tomorrow's Manpower Needs,* Vol. IV, rev. Washington:
Government Printing Office, 1971.

Vahovich, Steve G., ed. *Profile of Medical Practice, 1973.* Chicago: Center for Health Services Research and Development, American Medical
Association, 1973.

Ward, Richard A. *The Economics of Health Resources.* Reading, Massachusetts: Addison Wesley, 1975.

Wilson, Florence A., and Newhouser, Duncan. *Health Services in the*
*United States.* Cambridge, Massachusetts: Ballenger, 1974.

Yett, Donald E. *An Economic Analysis of the Nurse Shortage.* Lexington, Massachusetts: D.C. Heath and Co., Lexington Books, 1975.

# Index

# About the Authors

Harold M. Goldstein is Professor of Economics and Director, Center for Medical Manpower Studies, Northeastern University, Boston, Massachusetts. In addition, Dr. Goldstein is Senior Scientific Associate at Boston City Hospital, a member of the Health Planning Council for Greater Boston, and consultant in the area of medical economics to the Department of Health, Education and Welfare, the United Hospitals of Rome, the World Health Organization plus many other national and international health organizations.

Morris A. Horowitz is Professor and Chairman, Department of Economics, Northeastern University, Boston, Massachusetts. In addition, Dr. Horowitz is a member of the Labor Panel of the American Arbitration Association, Arbitrators Panel of Federal Mediation and Conciliation Service, and the Latin American Studies Association. He has been a manpower consultant in Brazil, Paraguay, Dominican Republic, Argentina, Spain and Italy.